OTHER TITLES OF INTER

AVAILABLE BY CALLING 1-800-MED-SHOP
OR BY VISITING HTTP://PMICONLINE.COM

OTHER TITLES OF INTEREST

CODING AND REIMBURSEMENT

Codelink® Guides to CPT and ICD-9-CM Code Linkages
Coder's Handbook
Collections Made Easy!
CPT Plus!
CPT & HCPCS Coding Made Easy!
E/M Coding Made Easy!
HCPCS Coders's Choice®, Color Coded, Thumb Indexed
Health Insurance Carrier Directory
ICD-9-CM Coder's Choice®, Color Coded, Indexed
ICD-9-CM Coding For Physicians' Offices
ICD-9-CM Coding Made Easy!
Medicare Compliance Manual
Medicare Rules & Regulations
Medical Fees in the United States
Reimbursement Manual for the Medical Office
Working with Insurance and Managed Care Plans

FINANCIAL MANAGEMENT

Accounts Receivable Management for the Medical Practice
Business Ventures for Physicians
Financial Planning Workbook for Physicians
Financial Valuation of Your Practice
Pension Plan Strategies
Physician Financial Planning in a Changing Environment
Securing Your Assets
Selling or Buying a Medical Practice

RISK MANAGEMENT

Behavioral Types and the Art of Patient Management
Law, Liability and Ethics for Medical Office Personnel
Malpractice Depositions
Malpractice: Managing Your Defense
Medical Malpractice: A Physician's Guide
Testifying in Court

DICTIONARIES AND OTHER REFERENCE

Health and Medicine on the Internet
Medical Acronyms, Eponyms and Abbreviations
Medical Phrase Index
Medical Word Building
Medico-Legal Glossary
Medico Mnemonica
Spanish/English Handbook for Medical Professionals

AVAILABLE BY CALLING 1-800-MED-SHOP
OR BY VISITING HTTP://PMICONLINE.COM

ACCOUNTS RECEIVABLE MANAGEMENT
for the
MEDICAL PRACTICE

Second Edition
J. Dennis Mock

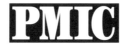

Library of Congress Cataloging-in-Publication Data

Mock, Dennis J.
    Accounts receivable management for the medical practice /
        Dennis J. Mock -- 2nd ed. p. cm.
    Includes index.
    ISBN 1-57066-213-4
    1. Medicine--Practice--Accounting. 2. Medicine--Practice--
Finance. 3. Accounts receivable--Management. I. Title.

R728 .M63 2002
610'.68'1--dc21

                                        2002035553

ISBN: 1-57066-213-4

Practice Management Information Corporation, Inc.
4727 Wilshire Blvd., Suite 300
Los Angeles, California 90010
1-800-MED-SHOP

http://www.pmiconline.com

Printed in the United States of America

ABOUT THE AUTHOR

Dennis Mock's background in health care receivables, accounts receivable management, and collections of delinquent health care accounts is extensive. He has taught classes for the American Association of Oral and Maxillofacial Surgeons; the American College of Emergency Physicians; and AMA Financing and Practice Services Inc., a subsidiary of the American Medical Association. He has been serving on an advisory committee for Medicare Part B, Illinois, since 1990.

In addition, he has served as the president of the Illinois Collectors Association, American Collectors Association, and the Medical-Dental-Hospital Bureaus of America. He is also a certified instructor for the education department of the American Collectors Association and has conducted numerous workshops throughout the United States, teaching professional debt collectors how to collect. He is also credited with helping start the first trade association for third party medical billers known as the International Billing Association.

Currently he operates a collection agency, Medical Business Bureau, which specializes in health care delinquencies. He does extensive consulting on accounts receivable management for physicians. He is also serving as executive director of Medical Dental Hospital Business Associates. Dennis and his wife, JoAnn, reside in Northbrook, Illinois.

DISCLAIMER

This publication is designed to provide basic, practical information on the subject matter covered. The information presented is based on the experience and interpretation of the author. Though all of the information has been carefully researched and checked for accuracy, neither the author nor the publisher accept any responsibility or liability with regard to errors, omissions, misuse, or misinterpretation.

CONTENTS

PREFACE

For the past forty years, I have had the wonderful opportunity of working with hundreds of physicians and their assistants on almost every economic issue that affects health care providers today. Although my expertise is in the billing and collection aspects of health care receivables, I also participated in the task of putting a value on practices for the purposes of divorce or sale. I assisted physician groups in the start-up stages by helping them find the financing, design a billing system, and negotiate outside contracts. I have served as a facilitator to several practices through the difficult times of closing down due to death or retirement. On a couple of occasions, I was directed by the courts to liquidate a practice. I also ran a billing company, which became the first electronic media claims submitter and for a period of time was certainly on the cutting edge.

Accounts Receivable Management for the Medical Practice is a compilation of the many things that I have learned during that forty-year period. The intention of this book is to pass on those lessons in health care receivable management to individuals in the medical profession. There are portions of this book that will hopefully serve as an aide, refresher course, problem solver, or guide for all members of the health care field: from the solo practitioner to the chief financial officer of a large multispecialty foundation; from the medical office manager to the receptionist. I have also come to learn that some of these ideas have tremendous value to bankers, attorneys, and certainly accountants. However, this book was primarily written for those individuals who have the desire and the responsibility to get the most cash out of a medical practice.

I began my career in this profession in 1962 when I joined an organization that was part of an unrecognized industry. Although in later years we would be identified as third party medical billers, we were also known in the health care arena as centralized bookkeeping or simply "those folks who bill the patients and collect the money." Today this business is called "accounts receivable management."

In the beginning, our billing company was targeted to a very defined market. Our principal clients were hospital based, and as a result we served as their "total office." With the aid of daily pick-ups or through the United States Post Office, on a regular basis we received what would best be described as the "encounter slip" which reflected the care the physician had rendered to the patient. Armed with this data, we billed the patient and completed any insurance forms. The money remitted was placed in the physician's bank account, and every thirty days we gave them a report showing the total charges and total collections, along with the total amount of monies still owed them, i.e., their accounts receivable. By the second or third month, if the patient hadn't paid, we were on the phone asking why not. If that didn't produce a resolution, we sent the unpaid accounts, which were few in number, to a collection agency.

This of course was pre-Medicare, pre-Medicaid, pre-managed care, pre-HMO, and pre-primary/secondary insurance. Looking back, the challenge was really more a matter of record management than anything else. Although Blue Shield as a form of insurance was becoming very popular, even that was relatively simple. With their red, white, and blue claim forms, a good typist could complete 20 an hour, because all of this was pre-automation. As a result, the ten-key adding machine was just as effective in determining the day's receipts. Of course, everything was simpler then. Today, although a few facets of medical economics have changed dramatically, most have changed very little or not at all.

The evolution of the way health care receivables are managed, including patient attitude, are part of my heritage. With proper management of your accounts receivable, you will have better control of your cash flow and be able to increase your profitability and provide a more economic stability to your practice. Although your primary concern will undoubtedly always be to provide appropriate health care services to the patient, you must do so in an efficient and economically sound manner in order to continue to stay in business services, especially with the current upheaval within the health care delivery system.

I sold the billing company several years ago for a number of reasons and now focus my attention on the collection of delinquent medical bills. In the process, I wanted to go back to my roots relative to that cottage industry and help it grow its own identity. The International Billing Association, now known as the Healthcare Billing and Management Association, was formed after a lot of work and with a lot of love. It allows those of you who manage multiple medical practices not only an identity but also a network to help you serve your clients in a more efficient manner.

It is my sincerest hope that the exposure that I have had will allow me to impart a number of ideas that will give some vision to the more successful running of medical practices. Although there are many aspects of this book that deal with "how to" and "how not to," many others should serve simply as excellent discussion points between practitioner and staff. Although health care and its economics are indeed going through numerous changes, it strikes the writer that some of the basic rules of thumb, now and in the future, will be usable.

J. Dennis Mock

CHAPTER 1

ECONOMIC EVALUATION OF A PRACTICE

An evaluation of the economic health of any business should include a consistent analysis of key figures, including as cash in bank, accounts payable, accounts receivable, and the relationship of key cost factors such as payroll and other expenses relative to the income of that business. A medical practice is no different. However, in evaluating a medical practice, whether it is a large group practice or a solo practitioner, one indicator should be analyzed on an ongoing basis because it can tell us more about the economic vitality of the practice than can be obtained from any other source: its accounts receivable (A/R).

Accounts Receivable Management

Accounts receivable, which is defined as the total amount of money owed to a practice for services rendered but not yet paid for, is an indicator of what is happening within the economic structure of a practice. As with almost any business, a medical practice should assess its economic health at least once a month. This is the single most important step in managing a practice's A/R. If done regularly and consistently, it will tell you whether a practice is growing or has become stagnant. Not only will you know whether there is a problem, in many cases you will notice certain signs that allow you to recognize situations and deal with them before they become problems. Equally important, this process allows a practice to set reasonable goals and expectations that are based on hard facts rather than on the perception of whether or not there is enough cash flow. Ultimately, it tells a practice if it is managing it's a/R or if the A/R is managing the practice.

A non-managed A/R, one that is out of control, can destroy the most successful practice. In a non-managed A/R, some assumptions are made. A practice renders the appropriate medical care to a patient and charges for it. The charge becomes an account receivable. The first assumption is that the patient or a third party on behalf of the patient will pay for that charge in a reasonable amount of time. Unfortunately, A/R involves not just one patient nor one charge, but hundreds of patients and charges. The assumed guarantor for the payment becomes an extremely diversified list of entities, each of which has created its own rules and regulations regarding when and under what circumstances the charge will be paid. Over a period of time, that list of receivables continues to grow, and although some of the entities will pay you, many will not. An A/R that is not managed can result in a situation in which an active, busy practice has insufficient cash flow to support its needs; it may not even have enough cash in hand to cover the payroll or even the phone bill.

Unfortunately, the A/R of a medical practice has little use other than to brighten a balance sheet as an asset. Accounts receivable do not create working capital unless they are collected. Most banks will not use them as collateral for a loan. A/R can be used in funding programs (programs where the A/R of a practice is "funded" by an outside entity) only if they are extremely well managed, which is not the case in this scenario. Finally, their actual value decreases as they age. A non-managed A/R with a value of $1 million can actually have a recovered worth, if aggressively pursued, of only one-quarter that amount.

Information Needed For Assessment Of Accounts Receivable

To perform the most basic assessment of an A/R, three pieces of information are necessary: monthly charges, monthly receipts and total A/R at the end of the month.

Monthly Charges

The charges for the month are the total amount of fees charged for patient care from the first working day through the last working day of the month, whether or not they have been paid. Charges for services that fall outside regular medical care should not be included. If you have been asked to testify as an expert witness and have just billed the defense attorney for $3,000, that is a charge and will undoubtedly produce income to you or the practice, but it should be considered outside income and for the purpose of analysis should not be included in the A/R.

Monthly Receipts

The second piece of required information is the total receipts for the month: the dollars collected for the medical care that was rendered. A receipt must always correlate with a charge that was entered for the current month or in a prior month. I remember a practice which had multiple sources of income, including rental space in a building it owned, book royalties and some significant income for equipment it had sold. Somehow this practice got into the habit of lumping the total income together. When they analyzed the practice's accounts receivable, the practice's owners used the income from all sources rather than from the medical practice alone. As a result, although their A/R management was deteriorating, it was not noticed for a lengthy period of time because the income figure was always substantial.

Month's-End Accounts Receivable

The third category of information needed to analyze a practice is the total A/R at the end of the month: the total balance that is due to the practice on the last day of the month for patient care. In reality, the total A/R should be the amount of money that can actually be collected eventually. Some factors can over-inflate this figure, such as failure to write off balances that are uncollectible. This could involve care for a homeless person who was not eligible for Medicaid or simply a regulatory balance (the amount disallowed by Medicare in accepting an assignment). Another way A/R can be inflated is by keeping accounts on A/R that have been sent to a collection agency. By turning them over to a collection agency, the practice has classified those accounts as "bad debt." For the convenience of posting collection agency payments, many practices fail to write off these balances or subtract them out of the total A/R. To perform a true analysis, it is essential that the A/R figure reflect the total money owed the practice which the practice plans to collect.

If one of these three pieces of information cannot be obtained without a lot of effort, the practice faces a significant challenge because this information is basic and, if missing, indicates a lack of receivables management.

Accounts Receivable Assessment

Once a practice has obtained the total monthly charges and receipts and the total A/R at the end of the month, it can begin assessing the state of the A/R. There are three methods of assessing A/R: days outstanding, A/R ratios, and aged A/R.

Days Outstanding

Days outstanding, or the average number of days it takes for a typical charge to be paid, is the method of accountability most commonly used by hospitals, and the same principles are applicable to a physician's practice. There are many ways to figure days outstanding. The simplest method is the following:

1. Take the accounts receivable of the practice on the first day of the month.

2.   Add to it the A/R of the practice on the last day of the month and divide by 2. This gives you an average of the A/R for the month.

3.   Divide this figure by the month's receipts and then multiply it by the number of days in the month.

The resulting figure gives you the average number of days a receivable is outstanding, or the days outstanding, for that month. For example, the equation below shows a practice whose accounts receivable on January 1 was $95,000. On January 31 it was $105,000, and the receipts for the month of January were $28,000. Worksheet 1 at the end of this chapter shows how to chart a practice's days outstanding.

EXAMPLE OF CALCULATION OF DAYS OUTSTANDING

$$95,000 + 105,000 = \frac{200,000}{2} = \frac{100,000}{28,000} = 3.57 \times 31 = 110.7$$

The average account is 111 days outstanding.

Influence of Financial Classes on Days Outstanding

An A/R can be categorized by financial class, or the type of financial arrangement under which the bill will eventually be paid, such as Medicare, Medicaid, commercial insurance, contractual care and self pay. The financial classes within an A/R vary from one practice to another and can have a great influence on the number of days outstanding. For example, in an orthopedic practice, the number of days outstanding is often much higher than is the case in other specialties. A large percentage of the receivables in such a practice can be categorized as "legal" because they result from accidents and can be tied up in litigation for months or years before they are paid. A practice with a large proportion of contractual care, such as a practice that sees patients under managed health care, can experience financial difficulties if the managed care organization is consistently late in its payments. There are other financial classes, including Medicaid, that have been categorized as slow to pay. If one calculates days outstanding on a monthly basis and puts that information on a graph, it will provide an indication of the direction in which the practice is going. Worksheet 2 at the end of this chapter can help you calculate the probable recovery rate for various financial classes.

What Should the Number Be?

The optimal range of days outstanding is 45 to 60. Normally this can be achieved only in a setting where accepting the payment at the time of service is commonplace. For a hospital-based practice, such as a radiology or anesthesia practice, 75 to 90 days outstanding is not a sterling example of receivables management but is considered acceptable. The real danger zone, whether the practice is hospital-based or not, occurs in practices in which the numbers exceed 120 days, unless there is a reasonable explanation such as a high percentage of Medicaid accounts. As a rule of thumb, any practice with 150 days or more outstanding faces significant challenges.

Accounts Receivable Ratios

Another method for evaluating a practice involves the use of A/R ratios. These ratios indicate how total A/R relates to a practice's payments and charges.

Accounts Receivable to Receipts Ratio

To find out how quickly your average account is being paid, simply do the following: Take the total A/R on the last day of the month and divide it by the total payments received during that month. Ideally this should produce a number ranging from 2.5 to 4. If the number is 5 or more, you are looking at 150 days (5 X 30 days) from the time when a charge is entered on the books until the time when it is collected. For example, if a practice has an A/R of $100,000 on January 31 and total receipts for the month are $30,000, the ratio of A/R to payment is 3.3, meaning that it takes an average of 3.3 months, or approximately 100 days, for a charge to be paid. Worksheet 3 at the end of this chapter will help you figure out you're a/R-to-receipts ratio and A/R-to-charges ratio.

EXAMPLE OF AN A/R-TO-RECEIPTS RATIO

$$\$100,000 \div \$30,000 = 3.3$$

The A/R-to-receipts ratio is 3.3

$$3.3 \text{ X } 30 \text{ days} = 100 \text{ days average for an account to be paid}$$

Accounts Receivable to Charges Ratio

It is possible to monitor a practice by keeping track of how the A/R relates to the practice's charges. Simply divide the A/R at the end of a given month by the charges entered during that month. For example, a practice with an A/R of $100,000 on January 31 and $25,000 worth of charges that month had an A/R-to-charges ratio of 4.

$$\$100,000 \div \$25,000 = 4$$

This number should be fairly consistent from month to month if there is good A/R management. It also should be somewhat similar to the A/R-to-receipts ratio. If the numbers vary dramatically, this may indicate that the practice is influenced by seasonal changes, as in the case of an orthopedic surgeon practicing near a ski resort. In the winter, the surgeon's A/R-to-charges ratio may be lower than it is in the summer when there aren't as many broken bones. Of course the A/R-to-receipts ratio also would be affected. Again, any number above 5 justifies a serious look at the practice's economic health.

Aged Accounts Receivable

A third method for measuring the economic health of a practice is applicable to practices that can divide their receivables by age into 30-day blocks. Most computer billing and accounting software allows you to break down receivables according to the month in which they were incurred. If the software cannot do this or if the A/R is not computerized, it can be done manually with some time and effort. Optimally, you are looking for an aging that, if charted, will form an inverted bell curve. This would mean that the majority of your receivables fall into the 30-to-60-day and 60-to-90-day slots. The inverted bell curve shows that you are collecting some charges at time of service and that you do not have an overload of delinquent accounts that are over 90 days. For example, a practice with a total A/R of $135,000 might have an aged A/R like the one that follows:

AGING OF RECEIVABLES FOR A TYPICAL PRACTICE

Age	Dollars Owed
30 days or less	$25,000
30 to 60 days	$45,000
60 to 90 days	$30,000
90 to 120 days	$20,000
120 and older	$15,000

If charted on a bar graph, these charges would look like Figure 1-1. However, if the A/R ratio is 5 or above, one gets a line that runs at a 45-degree angle from the first 30-day aging to the last 30-day aging, as demonstrated in the aged A/R below and in Figure 1-2.

AGING OF A PRACTICE'S RECEIVABLES WITH AN A/R TO PAYMENT RATIO OF 5

Age	Dollars Owed
30 days or less	$25,000
30 to 60 days	$30,000
60 to 90 days	$35,000
90 to 120 days	$40,000
120 and older	$45,000

Figure 1-1: Dollar value of aged receivables for a practice whose receivables are in line

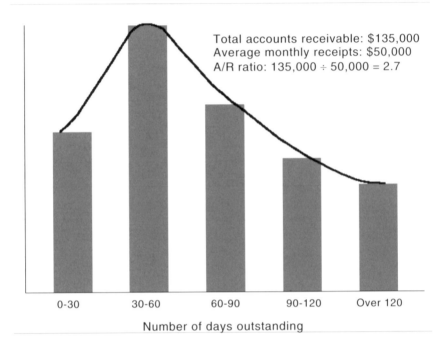

Total accounts receivable: $135,000
Average monthly receipts: $50,000
A/R ratio: 135,000 ÷ 50,000 = 2.7

Number of days outstanding

Figure 1-2: Dollar value of aged receivables for a practice with an A/R to payment ratio of 5 or more

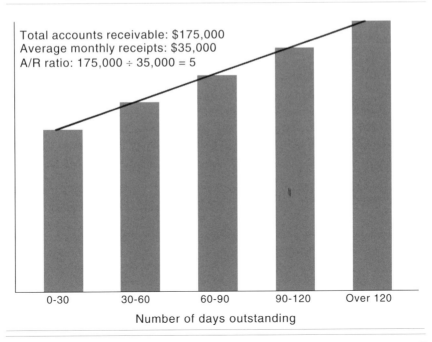

Total accounts receivable: $175,000
Average monthly receipts: $35,000
A/R ratio: 175,000 ÷ 35,000 = 5

Number of days outstanding

Distribution of Aged Receivables

The ability to age a practice's receivables is a critical element in A/R management, especially if one can age each financial class separately and identify how each one is performing. For example, there can be a big difference between the aging of commercial insurance and that of self-pay, the charge or portion of a charge for which the patient is responsible. When the aged A/R shows a mass increase in the percentage of accounts over 120 days, it takes a lot of effort to determine whether this is the result of commercial insurance accounts, self-pay accounts, or both. By tracking aging of the A/R by financial class, realizing that each class will have its own characteristics, you can be more accurate and efficient in spotting areas that need attention rather than attacking the entire A/R.

Many practice management experts strongly recommend that the distribution of receivables look like Table 1-1. As the receivables age, they should decline as a percentage of the A/R. This distribution of A/R aging may be idealistic for many practices, idealistic from the standpoint that there are contributing factors that the practice may not be able to control. It may depend upon the distribution of the financial classes of patients. For example, a practice with an extremely high percentage of Medicaid patients and an equally high percentage of slow-paying contractual care patients will not be able to achieve this distribution, whereas an office-based practice that collects from more than 50 percent from its patients at the time of service will have different norms. The practice must understand what is affecting the distribution and determine whether it is controllable.

I know of a practice that installed a new software system for its billing and A/R management. The employee who did the set-up had many options for fitting the system to that particular practice setting. One involved the length of the billing cycle. In essence, this was a matter of determining the number of months a patient would be billed before another action, such as collections, was taken. On the basis of the type

Table 1-1: Recommended Distribution of Accounts Receivable by Age

Age of Accounts, days	Total A/R Not to Exceed %
0 - 30	40
31 - 60	30
61 - 90	15
91 - 120	10
More than 120	5

of practice and the geographic locale, the employee thought that all patients would have paid their bills within four months and set the indicator so that at the end of four months that patient's entry item would no longer generate a statement. Her feeling was that there would be so few unpaid accounts at the end of four months that the situation would be manageable. For four months after the conversion to this electronic system everything seemed to be working quite well. Shortly thereafter, however, the practice noticed a significant increase in it's A/R and a reduction in its receipts. After about a year, it added a third practitioner, thinking that the increased volume would help overcome what was now becoming a crisis of cash flow. Initially, at least for four months, it appeared that this was helping to a degree. However, by the fifteenth month from the time of conversion, the practice was having difficulty making the payroll.

Everyone in the practice was aware of the increase in receivables, yet no one focused on the fact that every month the percentage of receivables over 120 days old was increasing steadily. By the time we became involved, only about 35 percent of the patients who owed the practice money were receiving a monthly statement. If the practice had monitored the distribution of receivables, it would have discovered the problem and developed a solution rather than just wondered why its receivables were growing.

In another example, a clinic got itself into a bind when one of the five principals decided that he didn't like the practice setting and wanted out. However, as the founding member, he was sole owner of the computer and software. When the employees realized that he would be leaving, it didn't take them long to comprehend that when he left, so would the computer. The employees, not knowing what the future would bring, simply stopped working the receivables and within three months, 40 percent of the receivables were over 120 days of age.

Although the recommended distribution of an aged A/R varies from practice to practice, there are some things we know for certain. Receivables over 120 days of age should be a constant or decreasing percentage of the total A/R. If one notes rapid growth in this area, it could indicate one of the following:

1. There has been a significant change in the way the mechanics of the practice are handled.

2. The dominant patient financial classes have changed.

3. The practice has acquired a contractual arrangement which is not working.

4. A major event, such as a significant increase in unemployment in the community or a natural disaster, has disrupted the economic stream.

Regression Accounts Receivable Analysis

Regression A/R analysis is a valuable tool that most practices do not use (Worksheet 4, at the end of this chapter). It basically charts the receipts and write-offs for a month and traces them back to the month in which the charge was incurred. The first group of columns (columns A through C) shows the total charges for a month, including the number of accounts and the average amount. Columns D through F show the amount of those monthly charges that have been collected in the current month as well as in the year to date, and also the percentage that has been collected. Columns G and H show the total amount and the number of accounts that were written off for that particular month. In a more technical version the charges may be broken into financial classes for each month with the same amount of tracking.

This type of analysis allows you to pinpoint the areas of you're a/R that have a lower collection percentage and focus on them rather than looking at the entire picture and to determine where the problems lie. This type of pinpointing can tell you at a glance which areas of receivables aren't being collected. Most third party collection agencies use regression analysis to track the accounts you place with them. This type of analysis is becoming more common in A/R management and is something I would add to my shopping list if I were looking for new software. Although it takes a lot of computer memory to generate, the new PC systems have that capability.

Seven Percent Rule

If a practice has a reasonable balance in its financial mix of payers and is performing in a reasonable fashion (statements are sent out on time, and insurance applications are filed in an efficient and accurate manner), a simple test can show where the majority of its income is coming from. First, take the receipts in any given month and trace them back to the month the charge was incurred. What you are doing is basically a regression analysis. You will consistently find that a practice receives seven percent or less of its total income each month from receivables older than 90 days. In many cases, especially when a large percentage of the A/R is older than 90 days, the practice spends 20 percent or more of its resources chasing what amounts to seven percent of its income. The 20 percent factor used in this illustration can vary dramatically from practice to practice. It can be as high as 40 to 50 percent if a practice allows that portion of the A/R to continually age without proper treatment.

Look for Alternatives

Some percentage of staff time is used each month in an attempt to control older accounts because practices look at the total A/R and try to collect as much money as possible. Although there is nothing wrong with that, a practice could operate more economically if it got rid of A/R that had aged beyond a given point, say 90 or 120 days, rather than continuing to bill and service it. The seven percent rule is a reminder to the practice that it should be looking for alternatives. If the A/R has grown to the point where hiring an additional full-time employee is necessary, one needs to analyze whether this will generate enough income to cover the person's salary. The need for additional personnel will undoubtedly occur if growth of the A/R is a result of practice expansion, but if that person is needed because the bulk of the A/R is over 120 days and produces little return, the practice should consider outsourcing for this portion of the A/R, which is discussed later in this chapter. I am not suggesting that these accounts should be thrown away or simply written off, but the practice should find a cost-efficient way to handle them.

An example of this occurred when a large and diverse practice in a specialized hospital changed its third party medical billing company. Within two months, one of the strongest recommendations made by the new biller was to transfer a significant portion of stale A/R to a collection agency specializing in A/R clean-up. The practice consented to the recommendation and a month later the results were incredible. Two months later the practice's receipts were the highest they had ever been and that was without taking into account the income generated from the A/R clean-up done by the collection agency. The general manager of that progressive third party medical biller said later that it was obvious that the practice had inherited an A/R from its previous biller that had reached the point of being unmanageable. The new biller's staff was trying to keep up with the back end of the A/R and not focusing on the front end—the new charges—where the income was. Once they were able to get rid of that segment of the A/R, their people were able to return to the jobs which produced real revenue, not $20 payments. Even more astounding, within 90 days of that decision, the income of the practice continued to accelerate upward because the A/R clean-up was producing much of the A/R.

The Black Hole

Professionals who are accustomed to handling accounts receivable often use the term "black hole." It is basically the same as the seven percent rule with a more simplistic approach. The black hole is the portion of A/R that has been around awhile, is stagnant, and has insufficient staff to manage it. The size of the black hole depends on the percentage of the A/R that is over 120 or 150 days of age. As the percentage increases, the A/R gets unmanageable because more and more energy and resources are spent trying to bring it under control. As a result, less attention is devoted to the front end of the receivables (the portion of A/R that is less than 90 days of age and more likely to be collected). This creates a vicious cycle. Accounts from the front end of the practice, which could have been collected in a timely fashion if enough attention had been focused on them, now flow through to the back end (the black hole) and the problem becomes increasingly unmanageable.

Fifteen Percent Rule

Another factor to maintaining the A/R is that no more than 15 percent of the total A/R can be in the last ageing bucket. If you bill for three months (90 days) then your last ageing bucket (120 days) should not exceed 15 percent of your total A/R. Remember that ageing should be from date of first billing, not service date. If it is, you will find it very difficult to maintain A/R ratios.

Why Accounts Receivable Ratios Get Out Of Line

There are many reasons why A/R ratios get out of line. Sometimes this results from external pressures over which a practice has no control, such as economic recessions and high unemployment. However, there are a number of other factors that affect the A/R and can cause problems.

Incorrect Information

One reason why A/R ratios may be out of line is incomplete or incorrect information on a large number of patient files. Because information is missing or erroneous, the practice must reallocate human resources to get the correct information and in the process it breaks the rhythm of efficient flow-through of data which delays billing. Having insufficient quality control over the initial data entry can cause problems months down the road, as would be the case with a Current Procedural Terminology (CPT) code that is not compatible with an International Classification of Diseases (ICD-9-CM) code, or with a CPT code that is simply incorrect. You would not know for 30 to 60 days that you've got a rejected claim.

Incorrect addresses and phone numbers or having a post office box for the primary address of a patient can cause delays. The patient may want his or her statements sent to a post office box, but if there is no response, you need an alternative place for contact. Lack of a phone number is critical not only to the control of an A/R, but also to exposure if you have a reason to recall a patient. I know of emergency room cases in which the patient was treated and released without sufficient demographic data, and then several hours later it was found that there was a misdiagnosis because of later test results. In all cases of which I am aware, even if there was no phone number, there was a street address where hospital personnel could go to inform the patient. You can imagine the dilemma if that had been a post office box.

Delayed Billing

Delayed billing can also affect a practice's A/R. If a practice ages A/R by date of service rather than date billed, every day a statement is delayed can make the numbers look worse. It is important to remember that there is a scale of diminishing appreciation for medical care: The greater the time between treatment and billing, the more difficult the collection process. A patient receiving a statement immediately after the service is more likely to pay the bill than the patient that receives a statement weeks or months later.

Written Credit Policy and Employee Attitude

Two causes for inflated A/R go hand in hand: the lack of a written credit policy and poor employee attitude. The lack of a written credit policy that is understood by the staff can cause serious problems in regard to the collectibility of A/R. For example, if a patient calls and explains to a staff member that he or she can't pay the entire bill at this time, your staff member may respond by saying, "Send what you can," rather than informing the patient of a written credit policy which stipulates the norm for a reasonable payment plan. Written credit policies are discussed further in Chapter 5.

Employee attitude has a great influence on how a patient feels about paying the bill. Your staff members need to have a global view of how their jobs and specific responsibilities affect the practice. They also need to be given adequate training and support (such items as a written credit policy). If this is achieved, the employee's attitude will show that the office is well organized and convey to the patient the need for immediate payment.

Payment Plans

A practice that has a large number of its patients (and therefore its receivables) on some form of payment plan can have its ratios thrown off balance. This situation normally is inflicted upon the practice by the patients, not at the request of the practice. In regard to healthcare costs, people generally believe that as long as they are paying something, everyone will be happy. As a result, practices need to have a specific payment plan either in a written patient brochure or through direct explanation to patients of their responsibility and what is expected before treatment. If a practice fails to do this, it often ends up with patients who elect to set up their own payment plans without consulting the practitioner's office.

Most practices don't have a defensive plan for situations in which a patient sets up his or her own payment schedule. For example, a good method of handling the situation when a patient tries to make a small partial payment is to immediately inform the patient that although the

$5 check is appreciated, it is unacceptable and if a payment plan is necessary, the practice expects at least X% of the balance owing each month. "X" has been used since regional differences and various practice objectives call for a different perspective. Also, the type of practice and the amount of the outstanding balance have a profound effect of what "X" should be. For example, if a practice says it expects 20% of the outstanding balance each month for the next five months and is trying to achieve a ratio of 3 on it's a/R, it already pushed that account 2 months over the goal. However, if the outstanding balance is $1,000 for an obstetric practice and the guarantor is unemployed, achieving a payment of even 10 percent may take some effort.

It simply makes good sense to have a written policy regarding payment plans to guide the staff since a certain percentage of these plans will undoubtedly come out of your overall attempt to control the total receivables. All too often when you have a procedure that requires each patient to be phoned at the end of 60 or 90 days for an unpaid amount, the patient's first response is that he or she cannot pay it all at once. If your staff members have been instructed about what is and is not acceptable, they'll have a much easier time dealing with the patient.

It is also important to understand that most patients will then assume that if a payment plan is created, you will send monthly reminders. Of course you can simply continue to bill the patient, but the patient and the staff have to understand the additional cost that is being incurred. In many cases, it would be less expensive and therefore more profitable to give the staff the freedom to lower the bill and collect it in one payment or two rather than stretch it out over 10 months with 10 additional statements, 10 additional envelopes, and 10 additional stamps. Although I've seen countless examples of patients who have paid off significant amounts with small monthly payments, as a rule of thumb a patient will default on at least one payment within 4 months. At best, there should be an understanding that upon the first default the account will automatically go to third party collection because your staff will not have the time to follow up on it.

Insufficient Knowledge

Insufficient knowledge of your aged A/R or an inability to interpret the knowledge available to you because of time constraints may also lead to an inflated A/R. Obviously, having the technology to do an aged A/R won't help unless you use the knowledge it provides. All too often a practice will equip itself with modern technology for handling A/R, and each month that wonderful printer will print out numerous management reports, including the aged A/R. The practitioner and staff have to learn that this is not just another document that has to be filed for the accountant at the end of the year, but rather a document that contains a tremendous amount of useful information for improving the economic health of the practice. If your practice has an aged A/R, use it. Better yet, if you can age your receivables by financial class or even if you have the ability to do regression analysis, be grateful that you have these tools.

Many practices still use some form of manual system, such as ledger cards. For the most part, manual ageing is impractical because of the time required to do it. In practices that have less sophisticated equipment, a little inventiveness can go a long way. If you are on a ledger card system, use colored tabs and replace them each month with a color indicating that the account is one month older so that when you want to separate out all accounts that are at 120 days of age or older, they will be readily identifiable. I have witnessed a number of mechanisms for identifying problem A/Rs, but the most unique was simply to measure the thickness of the ledger cards at the end of every month. My hat is off to the manager of that practice. At least there was an attempt to establish some control over the A/R.

Correcting A Problem Accounts Receivable

There are numerous methods available for correcting an A/R that has gone out of line. If you can identify and diagnose the cause, you will be in a far better position to determine which of these ideas can give you relief. Of course this entire book is dedicated to helping a practice manage its receivables, but first it is important to understand several things. Financial matters are personal and when things aren't going right, it is hard to discuss them with others. However, if you can overcome that mind-set, you will begin to accept the fact that there are a number of people who are a part of your "team" but are not on the payroll. More often than not, they are excellent resources to help you correct a problem A/R.

Billing Companies

I am personally convinced that, given any situation, a case can be made for the services of a third party biller. Generally, when a practice takes its billing in-house, it is due to a previous negative experience with a billing company. If they spent the time, they would find that the bad experience was because they did not make an effort to correct a problem with the relationship.

A classic case was a large medical college where each specialty chose its own biller. Some of them made great choices, others not the best. Early on, the college decided to track the performance of each of the twelve companies that were on campus. Each of the companies was having a mutual problem. The college required each department to use the same tax identification number. Therefore, as one would expect, each department often received the others' mail. In time, one biller stood out as the best because it served the most departments and was able to track its incorrect mail. As time went on, it did better and better

15

compared to the competition and the college decided that it should become the biller for all departments. Without changing the tax identification number challenge, this company soon ran into the same problem.

The purpose of a biller is to do the job better and more efficiently than an in-house system. The basic reason is that it assumes total responsibility for all the tasks and functions that a practice would be struggling with: systems, personnel, space and software or hardware upgrades for regulatory changes.

Conversely, some may find limited tax advantages, and prefer having internal control by taking a hands-on approach. My personal problem with this option is that, all too often, the medical practice doesn't go outside because it doesn't want to expose a third party to an eternal problem. I will never forget an experience where a CPA was struggling with a cash flow problem in a physician's office. After a lengthy period of time, he finally told the doctor that he must use a third party biller. The CPA recommended our company, and three months later we were meeting with the CPA. We explained that there appeared to be internal theft taking place on a daily basis. Our problem was that it appeared to be the bookkeeper, but we couldn't rule out the doctor either. When the CPA shared our concerns with the doctor, he lost the client. From time to time, we heard from other billers who handled the account; there were several because the practice changed billers every time this problem was suggested. It wasn't long before the IRS caught up with the doctor who said, "If the CPA didn't catch me, I figured a biller wouldn't. Otherwise, I would never have gotten rid of my in-house system."

Who, then, benefits from using a third party biller:

1. A practice that does not know it's a/R ratio and/or its total A/R.

2. A group in which the partners no longer trust each other.

3. A practitioner who has had an audit, who isn't sure about coding, or who doesn't have a voluntary Medicare compliance program.

4. A practice that can't document its practice income.

5. A practice that has either a net or gross collection recovery that it believes is below norm, and for which at least two billers agree.

6. A practice which has software or hardware that: cannot tell it what's happening; is malfunctioning on a regular basis; fails to meet regulatory changes; or does not provide audit trails.

The truth of the matter is that almost any practice should and could find multiple benefits from using a third party billing service, provided the service offers a level of "best standards." This, unfortunately, is where the problem lies. It's not that a practice doesn't need a biller, but rather the practice can't find a reasonable marriage, or worse the practice wants a marriage where it is dominant.

The information provided in this book will help you understand what is good A/R management for a practice. There are no current standards for third party medical billing, therefore you must have a strong understanding of what you want and what is a reasonable expectation. Then, if you decide to use a third party billing service, you can look for the perfect marriage based on the economics of your practice.

Collection Agencies

One of the most important resources in this area is the collection agency you currently use. The agency may have other products and services it would like to sell you to help clear up the problem, but it also has extensive knowledge. If you have used an agency for a long period of time, it should have a pretty good outlook on why your patients have become delinquent. Many times it will know you have a problem before you've identified it. Based on the age of the accounts you are referring, it may be able to tell you the debtors' reasons for not paying their bills. If the agency is having trouble locating debtors who are "skips," (where statements sent to a patient have been returned because the patient has "skipped town" or moved), it can tell you that you need better demographic information such as place of employment, correct home address and phone number, and Social Security number.

Practice Management Professionals

Numerous companies and individuals specialize in all facets of the economics of health care and the overall management of medical offices and practices. Often attorneys will specialize in handling the economic affairs of a practice. Accountants are the most common practice management professionals. In addition, some corporations will have practice management consultants who will come to the office to do a complete examination of you're a/R, office procedures and policies, and make recommendations for overall improvement of your office procedures. The best method of finding a practice management professional is to ask your peers. You can also contact one of the practice management trade associations for a list of people in your area who are qualified to assist you in the management of your practice. This is a good alternative if you are having a serious problem with you're a/R and you have tried everything else.

Software Vendors

If your system is automated, your current software probably has a lot of facets you are not using. Because of turnover in the office or inexperience and unfamiliarity, your staff may not be knowledgeable about the flexibility of your software. Obviously, software vendors make money selling software, but you would be amazed at what they can tell you about your practice based on the way you are using the software. Remember that the person who determined all the parameters for your billing system did this during the installation of the equipment and probably made as many as 200 decisions about what you wanted the computer to do at that time. If this took place more than a year ago, reevaluating the parameters can be a healthy exercise.

I know of a practice that was having difficulty with its receivables. It turned out that when the computer system had been installed a few years earlier, the practice manager assumed that by the fifth month all receivables of that age would have been disposed of, so she established a parameter under which the patient was not longer billed when a receivable reached 5 months of age. Two years went by before the practice manager became frantic over the massive growth in A/R with no collections. The practice finally discovered the problem and changed the program. In the next 2 months the number of outgoing statements increased over 100 percent. Of course, this created a tremendous public relations problem. It is curious that no one thought to question the process before it had gotten out of hand, but similar situations have occurred throughout the country.

Professional Societies and Trade Associations

Over the years, the majority of professional societies have taken the position that they should not get involved in the economics of their members' practices. However, some medical societies never took that position, and others have changed. Regulatory issues and the increase in managed care contracts have prompted these societies to become more active in the economics of their members.

For example, the American Society of Anesthesiologists, in conjunction with the Anesthesia Administration Assembly, produced both a handbook and a video on economic issues affecting anesthesia practices. It is a noteworthy source of information on what to look for in managed care contracts and other forms of controlled economic delivery. Hundreds of societies and associations function under the auspices of the American Medical Association and depending on your specialty, you may find a wealth of information regarding your peers' experiences.

Listed below are several trade associations and societies outside of the American Medical Association that you can turn to for advice and assistance. It should be recognized that there are many others, particularly CPAs and attorneys, who have developed a reputation for primarily representing physician practices for whom no association is listed.

American Collectors Association

American Collectors Association, Inc. (ACA), 4040 West 70th Street, Minneapolis, MN 55435, (612) 926-6547, John W. Johnson, Executive Vice President. This is the largest association of third party collection agencies in the world. It has a division headed by Ted M. Smith called the Healthcare Services Program which represents a number of members who specialize in health care collections and many of whom are also involved in diversified services such as precollect and early out systems.

Healthcare Billing and Management Association

Healthcare Billing and Management Association, Inc. (HBMA), 1550 South Pacific Coast Highway, Suite 201, Laguna Beach, CA 92651 (877) 640-4262. This association, formerly known as the International Billing Association, is comprised of individuals and companies that are involved primarily in third party medical billing. Most of them are also involved in various levels of consulting to medical practices. Although HBMA members' interests are primarily focused on A/R management, many of the members are leading experts on managed care contracts and the production of patient brochures for the practice and are knowledgeable about regulatory issues.

Medical-Dental Business Associates

Medical-Dental-Hospital Business Associates, Inc. (MDHBA), 1550 N. Northwest Highway, Suite 403, Park Ridge, IL 60068, (888) 751-0481. This is a small organization which was formed in 1932 by a few owners of collection agencies throughout the United States. Their initial stated purpose was to improve the image of the collection industry. In the process, the scope of activities expanded to diversification within the collection industry, and they are recognized as the founders of the concept of centralized bookkeeping and third party medical billing. Although the member's activities are primarily in the collection of delinquent accounts, A/R clean-ups and management of partial payment accounts, they are connected among themselves by a network of sharing and have consistently demonstrated leadership in the economics of health care.

Medical Group Management Association

Medical Group Management Association, Inc. (MGMA), 104 Inverness Terrace East, Englewood, CO 80112-5306, (303) 799-1111. This is an association of managers of medical groups. One of its activities is polling its large membership on a continuing basis. They can tell you the range of salaries for an office manager by region and specialty, along with the types of fringe benefits that should be associated with it.

National Association of Healthcare Consultants

National Association of Healthcare Consultants (NAHC), 1255 23rd Street, N.W., Suite 850, Washington, DC 20037-1174, (800) 313-6242. This trade association was formed in 1993 and represents a merging of several groups, one of which was the Society of Professional Business Consultants. The membership is comprised of CPAs, financial planners and enrolled agents. The members deal with the business side of a practice including legal issues, contracts and computer technology.

Suggestions from Peers

Recommendations from peers can be extremely helpful. After all, your peers are feeling the same economic and regulatory pressures you feel. However, I would strongly encourage the avoidance of locker room talk. Perhaps the best explanation of locker room talk is provided by a short story. I share this only because I am sure the statute of limitations has run out. In the early 1970s, my company's primary function was third-party billing, principally for hospital-based physician groups. From my vantage point, we were doing an incredibly good job and any loss of clients was due primarily to retirement.

I was taken aback one day when I got a phone call from a client who represented a very small group, basically himself and his wife, and was going to do his own billing. He explained in earnest how during the previous weeks he had observed in the locker room the outstanding surgeon of a newer hospital telling his peers some of the reasons for his economic success. Among them he mentioned a CPA-tax attorney and strongly suggested that this surgeon do his billing from his home. This was at a time when there were numerous tax loopholes for home offices.

When I talked to him several months later, he said it was working out quite well and he explained how he had both of this children on the payroll. I was somewhat surprised knowing that one child was four and the other was six. In theory it was a great economic idea and in all probability, even if he didn't do a great job on the billing, he would be economically ahead. I couldn't resist asking what would happen if the IRS questioned what his 4-year-old or 6-year-old were doing on the payroll. He calmly responded, "That's all worked out. They lick the stamps that we put on the billing statements."

Several years later I wasn't surprised to hear that he was spending thousands of dollars defending himself with the IRS. Shortly thereafter I read in the local paper that a judge had sentenced him to 90 days in prison to discourage other wealthy physicians from trying to beat the system. If it sounds too good to be true, it probably is.

Staff Input

Never overlook the value of your staff's observations. If you are convinced that there is a problem in the practice that needs outside help, ask your staff if they have a solution to the problem. Very often you will be surprised at their insight. That part-time employee who does nothing more than stuff statements into envelopes for the monthly mailing may be able to tell exactly what's wrong. Ask and listen. It can prove to be very beneficial.

The Office Supply Vendor

Another source of information is the individual who supplies your billing statements and envelopes. In most cases, he or she will be pleased to show you what other medical practices in your area do to make their billing statements more understandable and the types of messages they use to elicit prompt responses from patients. Although the vendor's specific service is to sell you a given product, if it is health care related you can assume he or she is selling it to more than one physician. He or she can share with you how other physician's practices are using that product to increase their efficiency. Even though many of the vendor's ideas will be based on its desire to sell you a specific product, this should give you and your staff a better idea of how other practices in your area are communicating with their patients.

Your office supply vendor can be a radar system for tracking what's going on in your area. Although this is not necessarily true in larger communities, a vendor who is close to the customers he or she is servicing, particularly in health care, will often know about individuals who are currently unemployed, looking for work, or about to leave a practice to seek a job in another practice. The same is often true of the drug or medical supply salesperson. Just finding a few minutes talking to a wider community of those who have interest in physician practices can prove very worthwhile.

Outsourcing

Outsourcing, or using a source outside your office for the management of all receivables over 150 days old, more often than not can be done by the kind of precollect system offered by most collection agencies. Another concept being used by many hospitals today is know as "early out" in which the receivables are transferred from the office to a third party very early on. The third party is given 30 to 45 days to collect anything and everything it can. This is a scenario that works particularly well for a practice that is growing rapidly and doesn't have the personnel to manage its receivables, or a practice that is cash-starved and needs to raise its cash flow immediately.

It is often desirable to outsource receivables that are on a payment plan to a third party such as a collection agency. Patients who are on a payment plan are those who owe a large amount and must pay on a monthly basis. There is often a lot of bookkeeping and patient contact involved. The agency is far better equipped to follow up and make sure monthly payments are made. All these services can be obtained on a contingency basis that is surprisingly inexpensive and in most cases costs less that what you are paying your staff.

Another method that is growing in popularity involves outsourcing tedious phone calls such as patient follow-up calls to see why payment hasn't been made and calls to self-pays. The collection agency usually can find a method to download these accounts from your computer to its computer and then put them on a system known as predictive dialing. Predictive dialing is a technology which allows the collector to make many phone calls in a relatively short period of time efficiently, effectively, and with a capacity that cannot be surpassed. If you're a/R ratio is at 7 with no reasonable explanation, a mere readjustment of your office staff will not correct the problem.

Of course there is a downside to outsourcing. The first, and the most readily identifiable, is the fact that if you elect to outsource any of your receivables someone in your practice will still have to act as the liaison and oversee it. If the time commitment for that function becomes significant, there is a good chance that you won't gain anything at all.

The second drawback is cost efficiency. Again, that requires monitoring from your staff, and unless clear parameters were set up in the beginning as to how that would be done along with an evaluation of the results of the outsourcing, this can become complex. For example, my company had the opportunity to offer a precollect program to a client which was run, as a test, on a first group of receivables. The results on the first batch of work were phenomenal. The results were so good that I was suspicious and told the client not to expect this every time. The client felt that even if our performance was only half as good as the next time, it would be well worth it. As a result, we entered into an agreement for a set amount so that even if the recovery on the next batch was only 50 percent, the client would still be ahead. As you probably have guessed, on the next batch of receivables and the batch following that, the results were not 50 percent compared with the first test—they were close to zero. Luckily, their organization and ours had the management skills to identify that problem, and as a result we modified our relationship. The point to remember here is that if you enter into an outsourcing arrangement, it will require continuous monitoring of the relationship to ensure that the desired results are being achieved.

Finally, it is important that the practice find time to research the company to ensure that it can fulfill the practice requirements. Many times that goes beyond determining the cost. For example, a collection agency rendering a precollect program still has to be in compliance with the federal Fair Debt Collection Practices Act (FDCPA). Certainly it is in your best interest that it do so, and if you have the slightest doubt about whether what you are doing is correct, it should be explored to the fullest.

The overall idea of outsourcing is to give a project or task to another entity that can perform it at a lower cost and a better rate of return than would be achieved if you continued to do it internally. Make sure that you have parameters that can measure the progress and the personnel to oversee it.

The New Practice

The information provided up to this point applies primarily to existing and established practices. If there is one area where expectations normally exceed reality, it is in a new practice. A new practice has greater needs because it is going through a learning situation with its personnel, patients, and environment. Although public relations are important in all aspects of health care, this is a much more sensitive area in a new practice.

A new practice also is faced with inexperience and lack of knowledge about things such as the payment reimbursement policies and time schedules of managed care organization. Although daily deposits are important to all medical practices, they are paramount in this situation. The most commonly asked question about a new practice is how long it will take to create some form of cash flow. Since there are many variations as a result of type of practice, geographic location, and how long it takes to get third party provider identification numbers, there is no single answer to this question. However, there are some rules of thumb. If the generally accepted billing cycle for your type of practice setting is three months, meaning that after the first statement the patient will receive three monthly reminders before getting the final notice, it will take one cycle plus one month before the cash flow to the practice is reasonably consistent or at its maximum level.

In addition, a new practice should see its first cash flow at about 28 days or less if it is utilizing any form of electronic media claim (EMC) submittal, even if it is only for Medicare. A practice should start to get some form of cash flow within 45 days, and then drop below that level for approximately 30 days if the billing is being done internally rather than through a third party biller. This is largely due to the fact that billing done on an internal basis traditionally gets done appropriately and in a timely fashion during the first days after the opening of a practice. Then, as the volume mounts, fine-tuning needs to be done in regard to staff responsibilities, among other things. More likely than not, a slow-down of the billing will take place for a brief period.

If the practice is using a third party billing service, the cash receipts tend to increase every week after 45 days. This assumes that there was sufficient lead time for the practice to secure provider codes and in many cases execute EMC agreements. Therefore, as a rule of thumb, new practices should have access to cash for at least 90 days of operation for payroll, rent and malpractice insurance before assuming that there is sufficient cash flow for third party vendors and a paydown of any type of loan that was created to start the practice.

There is a dramatic difference between new practices that are office-based and those which are hospital-based. An office-based practice that collects from its patients at the time of service is obviously in a much more controllable situation relative to its economic destiny than is a hospital-based practice. However, there are geographic areas where collecting at the time of service is frowned on and may not be done by a practitioner's peers. It is very hard to grow a practice if you are the only one on the block asking for payment at the time of service.

One alternative to this is to explain to your patients that you have implemented a relationship with MasterCard and Visa for payment at the time of service, recognizing that it will make things easier for them and for you in terms of saving on billing costs. The second alternative, which can be very attractive to the patient, is to offer a discount for paying at the time of service. Your justification would be the money saved in billing costs, which most patients will understand. If you look at your billing costs, almost any discount you are willing to offer could be justified. Within either of these alternatives, it should appear to the patients that you've made it easier for them rather than for yourself.

Finally, a lot of this can be achieved through creating a bond with the patient. For example, give patients a questionnaire with questions such as, "We've done our best to give you the highest level of medical services. How can we serve you better?" At the same time, tell your patients what you are doing to make access to your practice easier. Tell them that you're proud to introduce a system by which they can pay by MasterCard or Visa, or explain the rationale for giving a discount. Whether it's attractive to you or not, you are a service organization. Getting cookies at Christmas may not be why you practice medicine, but it is very important that your patients buy into your practice so that they want to support it and help you grow.

A hospital-based practice which receives all its income through direct third party billing will normally have a limited flow of cash in its first 45 days. If the practice plans to bill all patients a minimum of once a month for 5 months before considering any of them delinquent, it will have to wait 6 months before its income stabilizes. In any case, although using A/R ratios and aged A/Rs as methods for assessment will not work during the startup of a new practice, they can do much during its formative period to avoid pitfalls such as the absence of a written credit policy.

Summary

A successful practice measures its economic health on a monthly basis by objectively tracking the relationship between monthly charges, payments and total A/R, using A/R ratios, aged A/Rs and regression analysis. A successful practice is aware of the 7 percent rule, which states that a practice receives 7 percent or less of its total income from receivables older than 90 days. If too much effort is spent trying to collect this portion, a black hole develops as more energy and resources are expended to bring it under control.

A thriving practice has the ability to self-diagnose when problems are developing, and in this process it sets benchmarks and develops internal systems that allow it to conduct a balanced and objective analysis of it's a/R management. Several facets can be detrimental in the way a practice maintains its receivables: incorrect information on patient ledgers; billing that is delayed; lack of a written credit policy; poor employee attitude; absence of a policy on payment plans; and insufficient knowledge or the inability to interpret the knowledge that is available.

A practice that is actively aware of the resources it has at its disposal will be able to accomplish its goals more readily. Those resources include the collection agency, practice management professionals, software vendors, professional societies and trade associations, suggestions from peers, staff input, office supply vendors, and outsourcing to a third party.

The economic status of a new practice demands additional assistance in areas such as getting adequate cash flow, establishing policy for payment at the time of service and developing proper relations with patients. In this process, it has set benchmarks and developed internal systems that allow it to conduct a balanced and objective analysis of it's a/R management.

WORKSHEET 1
page 1

CALCULATING DAYS OUTSTANDING

Step 1: Calculate the average A/R for the month. Add the total A/R at the start of the month to the total A/R at the end of the month, and divide this figure by 2. This is your average A/R for the month.

Month	A/R at Start	+	A/R at End	÷2=	Average A/R
Jan.		+		÷2=	
Feb.		+		÷2=	
Mar.		+		÷2=	
Apr.		+		÷2=	
May		+		÷2=	
June		+		÷2=	
July		+		÷2=	
Aug.		+		÷2=	
Sept.		+		÷2=	
Oct.		+		÷2=	
Nov.		+		÷2=	
Dec.		+		÷2=	

Transfer the average A/R to column 2 of the corresponding month on page 2.

WORKSHEET 1
page 2

CALCULATING DAYS OUTSTANDING

Step 2: Calculate the days outstanding. Divide the average A/R by the monthly receipts. Multiply this ratio by the number of days in the month. The resulting number will be the average number of days an account is owed to your practice, or the days outstanding.

Month	Average A/R	÷	Monthly Receipts	=	Ratio	x	Days	=	Days Outstanding
Jan.		÷		=		x		=	
Feb.		÷		=		x		=	
Mar.		÷		=		x		=	
Apr.		÷		=		x		=	
May		÷		=		x		=	
June		÷		=		x		=	
July		÷		=		x		=	
Aug.		÷		=		x		=	
Sept.		÷		=		x		=	
Oct.		÷		=		x		=	
Nov.		÷		=		x		=	
Dec.		÷		=		x		=	

WORKSHEET 2

CALCULATING PROBABLE RECOVERY FROM VARIOUS FINANCIAL CLASSES

Total accounts receivable: $ _____

Financial Class	% of A/R	Dollar Amount	x	Probable Recovery*	=	Dollar Value
Medicare			x		=	
Commercial Insurance			x		=	
Blue Cross/ Blue Shield			x		=	
Worker's Comp.			x		=	
Contractual: HMOs			x		=	
Contractual: PPOs			x		=	
Self-pay			x		=	
Professional Courtesy			x		=	
Other			x		=	
				Total:		

Total dollar value divided by the number of months of your billing cycle equals your expected average monthly receipts:

$ _____   ÷   _____   = $ _____

Total dollar value   Months per billing cycle   Average monthly receipts

Probable recovery is based on your historical knowledge of the practice, input from peers and a sampling taken by grouping a number of payments from the same financial class to calculate that percentage. As a rule of thumb, you will find that the first four categories in this list are 80 percent, contractual care (HMO and PPO) is 60 percent, self-pay is 55 percent, and professional courtesy is 70 percent.

WORKSHEET 3

CALCULATING ACCOUNTS RECEIVABLE RATIOS

A/R to Receipts Ratio

Total of last 12 months'
     receipts: $_____ ÷12= $ _____
                                                  Avg. monthly
                                                  receipts

Total accounts receivable: $_____

$_____ ÷ $_____ = _____
   Total A/R   Average monthly   A/R to receipts
                   receipts   ratio

Scoring Guide	
2—3.5	Excellent
3.5—4	Good
4—5	Practice has some challenges
Over 5	Practice probably needs help

A/R to Charges Ratio

Last month's charges: $_____

Total accounts receivable: $_____

$_____ ÷ $_____ = _____
   Total A/R   Average monthly   A/R to charges
                   receipts   ratio

    If you do this for a 12-month period, you will see consistency in the A/R to charges ratio unless you have a seasonal practice. Optimal ratios are similar to those for A/R to receipts ratios.

WORKSHEET 4

FORMS USED FOR REGRESSION ANALYSIS

Date	CHARGES			RECEIPTS			RETURNS	
	Number of Accounts	Total Charges	Average Amount	Amount Received This Month	Amount to Date	Percentage	Number of Accounts	Net Amount
	A	B	C	D	E	F	G	H
Jan.								
Feb.								
Mar.								
Apr.								
May								
June								
July								
Aug.								
Sept.								
Oct.								
Nov.								
Dec.								

Formulas: $C = B \div A$ $F = 100 \times [E \div (B - H)]$

CHAPTER 2

SETTING GOALS

I agree with the concept that if you don't know where you're going, any road will get you there. When it comes to setting goals for effective A/R management, the problem is that you and I don't know each other. A number of things can affect the management of A/R: your relationship with your partners, your need to expand and market the practice, and your contractual relationships. Each practice is an entity unto itself, with unique goals and objectives. Although I may not know your specific problems and goals, I do know that numerous factors help shape our vision of our wants and needs. This chapter will set forth parameters for reasonable, measurable goals, recognizing that A/R management is the lifeline of a practice. Some of these ideas may be unreasonable or unattainable, and others will piggyback on broader concepts of practice management.

For example, I worked with a two-person practice that formed a partnership several years beforehand for all the right reasons. However, with the passage of time, the practice's goals and objectives changed and they became totally different. The partnership was formed when one physician could no longer handle the many demands placed on her by her patients and the needs of the hospital with which she was affiliated. She no longer wished to work 60 hours and more each week, and wanted relief from the stress. In addition, she came to recognize that she was not a businessperson, and the practice desperately needed someone with those talents. In essence, she was a well-qualified practitioner who simply wanted to render care.

The partner she picked was a likely choice: young, energetic, well-organized, willing to work extra hours, with a business background not always found in new practitioners. It seemed to be the perfect match. However, as the years went by, problems developed. When I was brought in as a consultant, the dilemma in this relationship could be found simply by analyzing the practice's A/R. The new partner, with his business sense, had entered the practice into a number of contractual care agreements which only continued to increase the patient load. He brought forth many progressive ideas on A/R management, such as requesting payment at the time of service, which the senior practitioner was reluctant to accept. Any patient walking into the waiting room would see a very successful partnership, but in reality their A/R was out of control.

Among other things, the senior practitioner would not authorize any form of outsourcing, such as third party collection services. Their management tools became dwarfed by their needs since the senior practitioner saw no need for technological investments. At the same time, the junior partner's love for managed care contracts grew weekly. The senior partner wanted to talk about semi-retirement; the junior partner wanted to talk about adding a third partner and an additional office. The business end of the partnership ended up in a head-to-head battle with no resolution. Each physician had different goals and couldn't seem to compromise. Each practice is different and has individual ambitions. When I make suggestions, I hope you can modify some of those ideas so that they will meet the needs of your practice.

Improve The Management Of Your Accounts Receivable

Improvement in the management of A/R should be your primary goal. However, we have not yet defined what "management" of A/R entails and how it can be improved. Accounts receivable management is the process of taking daily charges for serving patients and converting them to cash in the most cost-effective manner without negatively affecting the practice in regards to its contractual relationships, position in the community, and affiliations with peers. It is a balancing act to control the financial portion of a practice.

Although the term "cost-effective" is used in this definition, that does not mean that cheaper is better. If an individual appears at your door and says he or she can manage your receivables for a substantially lower fee, an evaluation needs to be done before you proceed. If the norm for A/R management in your area is 10 percent of income, which includes billing and collection, and someone offers to do the same thing for 5 percent, don't jump into an agreement unless you have all the facts, because it is probably too good to be true. You need to define what you want the outcome to be for the management of your receivables. I hope you will find the following to be reasonable and obtainable concepts for the overall goal of A/R management.

Involve The Entire Staff

The difficult side of managing A/R is monitoring the effects of your goals. You are busy with the medical aspects of the practice and must leave most of the financial considerations to members of the staff: office managers, medical secretaries, receptionists, billing clerks, and bookkeepers, among others. Keep in mind that no matter what your goals are, they will be difficult to reach unless you find a way to involve all the staff members in the process and get them to agree collectively that the goals are worthwhile and obtainable. Without that element, there is a good chance that you will get back fabricated information from staff members who are protecting their turf or showing their indifference.

All the staff members must understand how the goals will affect them and the benefits they will derive from achieving those goals. Therefore, before embarking on these steps, it's a good idea to look at some of the issues and procedures about which your staff may have already complained and now wishes to correct or improve. When those concepts are incorporated into the goal of improving A/R management, everyone has a chance to be a winner.

Staff Meetings

One of the most effective ways to start this process is with staff meetings, preferably on a set day and time, 52 weeks a year, regardless of who is available. This process is even more effective when a written agenda is distributed before the meeting. Staff involvement is more complete when there is a week-to-week rotation of the individuals who conduct the meetings. Numerous benefits accrue to an owner-practitioner who acts as an observer-participant at a meeting from time to time rather than running the meeting each week. Not only will it ensure that the meeting will be held regardless of who is available, it will give you a different perspective on how your staff perceives problems and their solutions.

Create an Agenda

The person who conducts the meeting should be the one responsible for creating the agenda. When you remove yourself from the role of running a meeting, you do not have to provide the agenda, and this gives your staff a chance to air problems they have observed rather than waiting for you to notice a situation and bring it up at a meeting. Depending on who is running the meeting, the agenda may focus on items that do not appear to be important to you but are important to your staff. The second benefit to having a staff member run the meeting is that it gives you a chance to back off of any new issue that arises if you need time to consider it further. If you didn't create the agenda item, you don't need to address it immediately. Probably the most important benefit of allowing staff members to run meetings is establishing the concept of a team. When all staff members participate, they become part of a team.

Assign Someone to Take Notes

Another key factor in a successful office meeting is to have someone record the notes. Included in the notes are any decisions that have been reached regarding policy, changes in work assignments, and the like.

By the same token, any topic for which a resolution was not reached should be added to the agenda for the next week's meeting or until a resolution is made. Notes should be taken on items the staff has collectively agreed need to be addressed further, indicating who is responsible for doing so. Meeting every Wednesday morning and airing the same problems will soon destroy the purpose of the meetings. Establishing a list of who is responsible for each topic for which a consensus has been reached not only will move the agenda item forward, but also will establish responsibility. At subsequent meetings the person responsible for each item should present a progress report. If a problem has been addressed for which there is no clear solution, it should be noted and addressed at the next meeting. These notes should then be typed, not necessarily in the form of minutes, but more to indicate who has accepted which responsibilities. Copies of the notes should be distributed at the next meeting.

For example, at the meeting of XYZ practice, the problem of excessive postage costs was reviewed. After much discussion, it was decided that the practice could save money by using a presort zip code service. Brenda volunteered to get additional information for the next meeting. If notes from the meeting included this incident and were distributed to all participants, it would be reasonable to assume that when they met next time, Brenda would have a report on presort zip code mailing costs and the benefits the practice would achieve by using that service. At the next meeting, it would be determined whether the practice would use the presort zip code service and who would be responsible for implementing it.

Provide a Progress Report

Along with notes from a meeting, you can also distribute a progress report for the practice. If part of the reason for the meeting is to review goals, a lot of time can be saved by having the information in printed form. This provides you with the added benefit of week-to-week or month-to-month tracking. Worksheet 5 at the end of this chapter shows such a form. Remember that you can change the form and include any information you are trying to assess on a weekly basis.

Find Time for a Meeting

A critical factor in scheduling a meeting is finding a time when there will be few interruptions. One way to achieve this is to set a maximum length of time during which you will meet. Initially you may feel that you can't cover everything, but over a period of time that will level out; even when you have only 20 minutes to meet, you'll be able to focus on the most critical issues.

Use An Erasable Marking Board

Another method that can be used to make weekly meetings more productive is to place a large erasable marking board in the room in which you meet (Figure 2-1). At the top of the board there should be two columns: "Good Things" and "Bad Things." If all staff members get into the habit of immediately going to the marking board when something good or bad occurs, this will form the nucleus of the agenda for the weekly meeting. If you use another segment of the marking board to post key numbers, such as A/R ratios, the percentage of receivables over 90 days, or whatever else you have targeted for improvement, this will serve as an effective tool for keeping everybody on the same wavelength and provide an ongoing reminder of how well the practice is performing.

Figure 2-1: What to display on the office marking board

Good Things	**Bad Things**
No insurance rejections this week	14 mail returns this week
No canceled appointments this week	

Target

Concentrate on getting better

Demographic information to decrease mail returns

Invite a Guest Speaker

Certain variations can be used to keep meetings interesting and informative for all the participants, such as inviting a guest speaker. Remember that your vendors, from the collection agency to the form supplier, can provide you with a tremendous amount of information about what's going on in their industries and what they see happening in your locale. They serve not only you but your peers as well, and are normally well versed on changes in the industry. For example, they can tell you any expected changes in the CMS-1500 form which is currently used for Medicare claims. They'll know when the changes will occur so you'll have a good idea about how large an inventory of CMS-1500 forms to maintain.

Your collection agency can keep you well advised about any changes in state regulations with regard to collection procedures. Since these regulations can be very complex, and are crucial to your practice management, having a speaker who is well-versed on the topic would be a smart move. More important, it can help keep your staff up to date on any potential obstacles to you're a/R management.

Maintain a Positive Attitude

It is important to maintain a positive attitude during meetings. One way to do this is to hold the meeting at lunchtime on occasion and provide lunch for all the employees. Even though your staff members may be asked to deal with some negative items, this will provide a positive aspect. If the practice has enough employees, a contest for the best idea of the month can do a lot toward getting staff members to participate and look for the positive rather than the negative, such as complaints about working late, the dress code, or personality conflicts. Although negatives will come, they often stimulate the staff's concern about employment and responsibility. If the practitioner is willing to react to those criticisms and specify how soon correction of a problem will take place, there will be increased bonding between the employees and the practitioner.

Don't Allow The Meeting to Become a Gripe Session

Although it is critical that your staff use this time to resolve outstanding issues, the meeting must not become a gripe session. Therefore, when a challenge is presented, make sure that a course of action is decided on and assigned to an individual for implementation or resolution. There is nothing more defeating than a small problem that crops up week after week without being resolved. One problem could be complaints from the front desk staff that they do not have time for a 30-minute lunch break. The morning appointments are constantly running over, and the afternoon patients show up early. If this problem comes up week after week at a meeting, it can get very trying. Simply confront the problem and make suggestions for a solution. One solution would be to lock the front door and post a sign saying, "We'll be back in 30 minutes." Another solution would be to occasionally take staff members to lunch or better yet, have lunch brought in. Once the employees realize that you are aware of the problem, even though no permanent resolution has been found, they will stop complaining if they get some reassurance that you really do care.

Another small problem that may occur from time to time is a complaint about dirty coffee cups in the lunchroom sink. It is detrimental to a meeting to have to listen to complaints as trivial as this every week. A good solution would be to have coffee cups made with the name of the practice on one side and the individual's name on the other side. At the end of the day, one glance at the lunchroom sink will indicate which employee(s) failed to rinse his or her cup and put it away. A couple of reminders to those people ought to take care of the problem.

Be Willing To Make Changes And Take Action

When you set goals and resolve problems, realism has to be your focal point. An aspect of that realism is that you have to be willing to make changes or take some form of action. For example, a few years ago we realized that an HMO was in serious financial trouble. We informed all our clients, but unfortunately because of various contractual relationships, they continued to treat patients from that HMO. Although I understood why they did this, the end result was overwhelming. Six months after we sent out the warning letter, the HMO went into bankruptcy court, leaving my clients with over $750,000 in unpaid claims. It is easy to understand why this occurred, but I still feel that when a red flag goes up, the practitioner should be in a position to take some defensive action. Perhaps the end result could not have been avoided, but we could have reduced the risk substantially by setting up weekly meetings with the HMO's representatives. Although at that time the state insurance commissioner was not overseeing HMOs, collectively we certainly could have done something to have an impact on the state legislature.

There are other examples where making a change is necessary. Let's take the goal of reducing insurance rejections. After some review, it is generally accepted that the rejections are high because the staff has had insufficient training in coding or completing the forms. Stating a goal and doing nothing about it will only add to the frustration. The practice has to be willing to make changes such as providing time for staff members to attend seminars that teach these techniques.

The problem of excessive staff turnover can also be a crippler to effective A/R management. If the practice sets reduction of turnover as one of its goals, it may have to increase compensation or add fringe benefits to resolve it. Another resolution is to hire an extra individual who is cross-trained in most job functions; this can help eliminate any gap when turnover does take place. If you set a goal, a road map has to be designed that is based on the conditions that exist within your practice so that you and your staff can see a way to achieve that goal.

Specific Problems And Goals

A number of problems and issues can affect A/R management; a few are listed below. Included with them are some basic goals that will improve your management of A/R, along with ideas on how to monitor those goals.

Number of Open Accounts

Although it is easy to understand why the dollars in you're a/R have to be managed, another factor that is rarely discussed is equally critical:

the number of open accounts. Every open account poses the possibility that a staff member will have to take some sort of action, whether answering an incoming phone call, sending out a monthly statement, or making a decision about what to do if it becomes delinquent. Even though there is a relationship between the number of open accounts and the size of A/R, people tend to forget that the size of the staff is often a reflection of the number of open accounts, whether those accounts are producing revenue or not. Every open account requires some form of monthly maintenance, such as generating a statement or answering a patient's inquiry. Therefore, as the number of open accounts increases in your receivables, your staff size must increase to give the proper amount of attention to the monthly maintenance. An A/R with 200 accounts needs fewer individuals handling it than an A/R with 2,000 accounts, even though the dollar amounts of each A/R could be approximately the same.

I realize this sounds extremely basic, but let me share with you the story of one practice. Although the practice had grown in size, it refused to add personnel. Not only did the black hole syndrome accelerate, the existing staff started to implement procedures for survival. One of the more unusual was to bill half the alphabet on alternating months. The rationale was quite simple. First, the number of statements per month had grown to a point where the staff found it difficult to get them in the mail. More important, they had fallen so far behind in all other office procedures that whenever the statements went out, it produced an influx of incoming calls from distraught patients asking why their insurance hadn't been filed, why insurance review hadn't been completed, or why refunds hadn't been made. Although the ratio of staff to open accounts varies dramatically with the discipline of a practice, if the A/R clerk once was responsible for 500 accounts and now is working with 1,000, the level of performance won't be the same even if the practice has advanced technology.

There is a significant difference between open accounts and active accounts. An open account is any account that still has a balance owing. An active account is an open account that has had recent activity and a strong possibility of being paid in a short period. Obviously, if there are few open accounts, your staff will have time to attend to all of them. However, if there are many open accounts, the seven percent rule mentioned in Chapter 1 is critical here. Many practices could achieve dynamic improvement by simply weeding out all accounts that have had no payment activity for the previous 60 days. This would reduce the inventory of nonperforming receivables and allow a greater focus on revenue-producing receivables.

My company has established a norm that no more than 5 percent of receivables should be over 120 days old. Obviously there are variations, but let's say you're a/R-to-payments ratio is 8 to 1 and, as a result, 48 percent of your receivables are over 120 days of age. In most cases you would be better off immediately writing those accounts off as uncollectible and giving your staff time to breathe. In all probability, the next month's receipts will show a significant improvement even though you have downsized your inventory. Although this may seem to be a paradox, your staff will be able to concentrate on current, active accounts which are more collectible, resulting in the collection of a higher percentage in a shorter period of time.

Mail Returns

It would be nice if every time you mailed a statement to a patient, it got there. Unfortunately, for a variety of reasons, that's not always the case. If this is an infrequent occurrence in your office, that's great. However, if it is common, it is a sure sign that other functions in the office are not performing as needed. In any practice, mail returns are costly. Let us examine several reasons why patient's monthly billing statements are returned and the effect mail returns can have on a practice.

Common Reasons for Mail Returns

Patient statements may be returned during the monthly billing cycle for any of the following reasons:

1. A/R may have aged to a point where patient mobility has caught up to it. It is estimated that 25 percent of Americans move at least every six months. Therefore, it is generally safe to assume that the older the receivables, the greater the number of mail returns. This process accelerates if the practice does not use the words "Address Correction Requested" on its outgoing envelopes. It is possible that the patient moved shortly after receiving the forwarding service. You received no mail return because the mail was forwarded to the patient at the new address. By the time you got that first mail return, the 6-month forwarding order had run out. Not only does not mail not get forwarded, you have lost the benefit of getting an address correction from the post office too. Even worse, the patient may have been making repeat visits without anyone updating the demographics on file.

2. Demographic information may have come from a source outside the practice, such as the hospital admitting office, over which the practice has little control.

3. Mail may have been returned because of a clerical error.

Addressing the Problem of Mail Returns

Whatever their cause, mail returns must be dealt with. In setting goals for this problem, you may want to consider charting your mail returns. First, determine the average number of monthly statements returned and, if possible, break them down by type or cause. Next, chart them on a daily and a monthly basis on a large billboard. Place the chart in an area where it can be observed by the staff daily. After doing this, you will be better able to pinpoint why mail returns are occurring, and as you address those areas, you will know whether this is having any effect on the number of mail returns.

I recognize how simple this sounds, but think about the costs and benefits. A mail return may represent a total loss of a receivable. In most cases your staff does not have the time, resources, or training to keep up with mail returns. Sometimes more time is spent trying to correct the problem than the receivable is worth. In essence, a mail return is an indication of a loss of a receivable that would have represented cash flow if certain things had taken place. Therefore, the practice will experience positive benefits if it simply assesses the following:

1. Accountability: Why is this occurring, and who is responsible?

2. Discovery: If a source for the majority of the mail returns is discovered, you and your practice can correct the problem and achieve better A/R management.

3. Improved income: Obviously if a patient doesn't receive a statement, there is little chance that the receivable will be paid. If the practice can reduce the number of mail returns, its cash flow will increase.

Insurance Rejections

Another goal you may want to set is to reduce the number of insurance rejections. Here you can employ the same process you use for mail returns; that is, you can chart the numbers and types of insurance rejections. First, categorize the reasons for returns. Categories to consider include wrong address of the insurance company, wrong procedure code, and missing or incorrect information.

Once you have identified the problems, you can become creative about reducing the number of rejections. After charting your insurance rejections by type, you may find that your office needs to adopt a policy of photocopying all beneficiary insurance cards and attaching them to the insurance paperwork. Depending on your specialty, you may find that it is essential to attach hospital records to your claims for certain Current Procedural Terminology (CPT) codes, the numbers assigned to specific medical and surgical procedures for universal identification. In other cases you may simply need to tell patients that, because of your experience with certain carriers, you have to request payment at the time of service. This puts the onus of dealing with the insurance carrier back onto the patient.

You may find that because of your rejection rate, phone verification is essential for your type of practice. If you find this suggestion too obvious, remember that if your average insurance turnaround time from point of submittal to reimbursement is 30 days, every rejection adds another 30 days to an account's number of days outstanding. The same scenario is true for managed care if the practice has not taken time to follow the mandated rules for the coverage and for a federal program such as Medicare or Medicaid if the practice has been unable to determine whether the coverage was in effect on the date of service. In many cases, a large part of this problem could have been eliminated by means of phone verification of coverage. Although extremely time consuming, this is one way to reduce the problem.

Incoming Patient Phone Calls

Except for the benefit of positive public relations derived from handling questions about billing and the opportunity to update information, there is no greater time robber for a practice and staff than patients' calls regarding their accounts. This type of call normally causes a confrontation, is upsetting to your staff, and doesn't help you collect the bill any sooner. You might consider tracking the types of calls your office receives, particularly as they relate to billing. You may find out something important in the process, such as the following:

1. Your current billing statement wasn't clear in giving the patient specific directions about what he or she was supposed to do. Through a relatively simple modification in software or a change in the wording of your billing statement, you can reduce those calls.

2. The patient didn't understand your fees or, more important, had a question about something that could have been clarified in the office at the time of service.

3. The caller didn't understand your credit policy because you didn't give him or her a practice brochure.

4. There was a clerical error.

Reducing the number of incoming phone calls, particularly when they relate to billing, not only will give your staff more time to handle other important matters, it will indicate that your practice and its patients are on the same wavelength. In essence, a well-run office is one where there is a full waiting room and incoming phone calls are made only for appointments.

No-Shows

If no-shows are an ongoing problem, the practitioner needs to get tough. One method for dealing with this is to give a staff member the task of calling each patient 24 hours before his or her appointment for confirmation. Some offices charge patients for broken appointments. The implementation of charging for broken appointments has some negative implications however, similar to the implications of adding interest or a service charge for slow-paying accounts. To what degree are you going to pursue the patient for collection?

One might consider some more imaginative alternatives. In one very busy practice, once the patient is identified as a probable or habitual no-show, he or she is no longer given appointment times. The patient's name is put on the appointment schedule in a separate column with the understanding that he or she will be fitted in, if possible. Another alternative for a habitual no-show is to always give the patient the last appointment of the day. Then if the patient appears, it doesn't interfere with the overall scheduling, and alternatively if the patient does not arrive, it has no negative effect on the schedule.

I tend to discourage charging for no-shows because invariably there is another side to the story. How often was the patient kept waiting for an excessive period of time? Or even worse, how often did the patient arrive to find that the doctor was tied up in surgery and would not be able to see him or her that day? In my mind, an increase in the number of no-shows not only has a negative economic impact on the practice, but also is a silent communicator of a relationship problem between the practitioner and the patient. Invariably, an increase in no-shows tells you that something else is brewing in the practice.

Continuing Treatment Without Noticing Delinquency

One of the most difficult problems in a busy practice is finding a way to deal with patients who have old unpaid balances yet continue to make appointments. Ideally, when you put a delinquent patient's number on the computer, the screen should flash and bells should ring when they call to make an appointment. Even though this happens in some settings, it doesn't eliminate the problem. Part of the problem is not having a written policy on what you will and will not do. Another part is that if the office is busy, no one may check the computer screen when an appointment is made. The third part is that for many practices, it is easier to make an appointment than confront the problem. Continuing treatment for delinquent patients may not be the worst thing that ever happens, but it represents the loss of an opportunity to collect a receivable and is a sign that other things may not be going right in the office, such as proper training so that the staff knows what to do in this situation.

Failure to Bill for All Charges

I work with a large residency program that believes it could be failing to charge for as much as 25 percent of the services it renders yearly. Quite simply, this has occurred because under the current system there is no incentive to turn in "encounter" forms or charge tickets. Although an encounter form varies from practice to practice, its primary purpose is to allow the practitioner to document the services that were rendered. Whether the form is 4 by 6 inches or 8½ by 11 inches is immaterial and more often than not is dictated by the needs of the practice. What is important is that it serves as the audit trail to explain why the patient is being charged. It is backup documentation for third party claims and is also a vehicle that can highlight many policies that an office-based practice finds desirous.

Traditionally the form is multipart with one copy becoming part of the patient's medical record, the second being used for posting charges and receipts, and the third copy going to the patient. It actually serves as the patient's bill at the time of service. In many cases it will contain additional information so that the patient's copy can be used by the patient to file for insurance payment. The policy highlighting can be achieved by simple statements or questions such as "Has your address or home phone changed since your last visit?" and "Payment at time of service is appreciated. Please note that we accept Visa and MasterCard." Encounter forms are an intricate aspect of the practice, but they can also be a creative part of the practice. They can be designed so that they take a minimal amount of time by using a checkoff list for standard procedures in the office.

However, for encounter forms to be effective, they must be monitored. If the second copy doesn't get to the accounting desk, the charge will be lost. In a smaller practice that can be easily overcome by simply balancing the number of patients seen with the number of encounter forms for the day. Even if the service was a recall or follow-up for which there was no charge, there should be an encounter form denoting that. The number of encounter forms and the number of patients should balance each day.

In multipractitioner and busier practices, the concept of prenumbering encounter forms should be considered. Although it may sound like an additional task and a lot of extra work to keep track of prenumbered encounter slips, let me tell you what happened at that residency program. Although the caseload of the department was increasing daily, many times involving as many as 200 patients a day, the gross charge dollars continued to get smaller. Even though the practice had a monitoring system for the charge tickets, as the practice grew, the procedure was eliminated because the front desk couldn't keep up with it. In addition, it was possible for a patient to see several physicians during one visit, and although the practice could allocate the charge ticket to the first physician, it was a nightmare tracking the slip once a patient left the primary physician. More important, in this setting many patients were seen by residents who had no concern about the economic side of the department.

The end result was that more and more encounter forms were not getting back to the front desk even though more patient care was being rendered. The problem was finally corrected by prenumbering encounter forms, signing them out to each practitioner in batch increments, and monitoring their return to the accounting desk. Although this required additional personnel, those costs were easily covered by capturing the charges for all services rendered. Although this system cannot ensure that a patient will be charged for all the services on the charge ticket, it ensures that some charging takes place. This is an area that both the practitioner and the staff should monitor.

Delinquencies

If you are able to age your total A/R in 30-day increments, one of your goals should be to reduce the percentage of cases that are aged beyond 90 days. When you get down to it, the reason you have a patient who has owed you for more than 90 days is that some of your staff members have failed. Therefore, if you set a goal of reducing this number, there is a good chance that everybody on the staff will become a team player; in all probability, each of them participated in the failure.

There are delinquent patients who are beyond the control of your staff. The most probable causes of delinquency usually occur during the first visit. Your staff might have failed to get complete demographic information, such as a copy of the insurance card, the phone number of the insurance company, and the patient's daytime phone number. Perhaps someone failed to explain the practice's credit policy before the patient was seen. Even though it is your policy to ask for payment at the time of service, perhaps no one did. Maybe a receivable became delinquent because the bill and the insurance claim were not filed on a timely basis or there was no phone follow-up to the patient or insurance company. Although you cannot prevent some patients from becoming delinquent, for many of the reasons mentioned in Chapter 1, there is a lot your staff can do to reduce the number.

Monitoring The Accounts Receivable Payment Ratio

Following A/R payment ratios is an important step in improving A/R management. This is probably the biggest indicator of improvement if the other goals recommended in this chapter are achieved. At the same time it will tell you other things about your practice.

Let's assume that you know you should ask for payment at the time of service but haven't been doing so. By monitoring the A/R payment ratio, you will be able to see whether a new policy of asking for payment at the time of service has been implemented by your staff.

Another benefit of this type of monitoring is that when you instruct a portion of the staff to do delinquent phoning, it gives you an indicator of the effectiveness of their phone calls. Finally, you can use this indicator to tell you whether you've improved the cash flow of the practice.

Monitoring The Accounts Receivable Charge Ratio

Monitoring the A/R charge ratio can and should be part of your overall road map to improving A/R management. Its purpose is more subtle and sophisticated than that of other indicators. The lower the ratio, the cleaner you're a/R will be in terms of eliminating a large percentage of accounts that are over 120 days. More important, lowering the charge ratio is a definitive indicator of any time lag between the date when the service was rendered and the date when the patient is charged for the service. This activity can do a lot in a short time to increase your cash flow and improve all the other indicators.

Consider that every day of lag from the date of service to the point when the statement is issued costs approximately 0.05 percent of the collectibility value of the account for the next 30 days. Therefore, during a five-day lag from the date of service to the date when the insurance claim is filed or the patient is billed, it is costing you approximately 2.5 percent in the form of a collection deficiency. This number can become enormous if the practice is fee-for-service hospital-based, in which case delays of 15 days or more are common. By reducing this lag time to zero where possible, one can achieve immediate returns on a significant number of these accounts. Obviously, some specialties can't avoid this time lag, but they should keep it in mind when setting goals. The importance for your staff of being part of this process cannot be overemphasized. There must be a method in place that allows you to monitor the days from point of service to point of bill. This probably should be added to the weekly monitoring chart.

Offer Incentives For A Job Well Done

Other aspects of goal setting may be helpful to your practice. Even though you may have established weekly meetings and created a team that is attacking new problems and eliminating old ones, you should consider whether compensation for the key players in your practice should be part of this process. Obviously, if the individuals who are responsible for reducing days outstanding lower them by 20 or more days, there is not only a direct economic benefit to the practice but a tremendous amount of savings as well.

Recognition of this success does not necessarily have to take the form of monetary compensation. A half-day off, a gift certificate or a special cake can tell the staff that you are willing to reward success. This is one of the more difficult areas to monitor, but if you write quarterly reviews of each targeted area to establish whether the goals have been met, you will be able to recognize the individuals who are directly responsible for meeting the goals.

Develop A Patient Survey

Consistently acting as judge and jury may not always supply you with all the information you need. Well-tailored patient surveys can draw out a different set of perceptions of how your practice is doing. Patient surveys are a science unto themselves and are most often considered when a practice is considering a major change, such as relocation to a different site. The practice tries to capture the patients' attitudes toward such a change before it is made. Since the economic impact of such a change is potentially significant, it is best to bring in people who specialize in that area of practice management. In a less sophisticated arena, such as new patients, one might want to consider enclosing a survey card with return postage with the first statement for new patients. This survey may ask simple questions such as "Was the office easily accessible by public transportation?" and "Did you find parking convenient?" or include an open-ended statement such as "We hope you enjoyed your first visit to our office. If we did not serve you in any way, please let us know." What you are trying to do here is look at your practice through your patients' eyes. You may be surprised at what they see.

Use Your Collection Agency As A Barometer Of Success

Many barometers can be used to measure the overall economic health of a practice. The following is applicable not only to office-based practices, but to hospital-based services as well. Let's say you and your staff have set up some definitive goals, such as reducing the number of mail returns, minimizing third party insurance rejections and capturing better demographic data at the time of service or first visit. In a short period of time you will notice that the practice's cash flow has improved significantly. However, there is another way to measure how successful your practice has been in meeting its goals. Simply look back historically to see what your collection agency has been recovering.

For example, if you've been turning over $1,000 worth of delinquencies every month for the last two years and the collection agency has consistently collected $300 every month, that's a 30 percent recovery. If you have set goals and have been successful in achieving them, the amount of dollars turned over for collection should have decreased. You should also note a net decrease in your collection agency's recovery percentage. However, if the rate of recovery continues at 30 percent, you either have the greatest collection agency in the world or some facet of your game plan is not working.

Summary

Managing A/R is a juggling act. You want to receive payment for the services you have rendered but you want to do so in the most cost-effective manner without negatively affecting the public relations of your practice. The best way to improve the management of A/R is to set goals and monitor their outcome. Not every goal can be achieved totally, but ongoing devotion will certainly lead to improvement.

Involving your staff in the goal-setting process can be to your best advantage. If staff members participate in this process, they are more likely to acknowledge that the goals are worthwhile and obtainable. Conduct regular staff meetings, using a written agenda, and keep track of your goals and accomplishments. Allow staff members to run the meeting from time to time or invite a guest speaker. Make sure there is written verification of any decisions or problems that have been brought up and assign an individual to follow through on them.

Some goals to consider include reducing the number of open accounts, decreasing the number of mail returns, reducing rejected insurance claims, controlling the amount of incoming patient calls, confronting patients who do not show up for appointments or have become delinquent in paying their bills, and making sure all charges are billed.

Once goals are established, be willing to make changes. Recognize the individuals responsible for achieving goals through some form of reward or incentive. Monitor the benefits of accomplishing goals by identifying changes in you're a/R payment and charge ratios, distributing a patient survey, or noting a net decrease in your collection agency's rate of recovery.

WORKSHEET 5

WEEKLY PROGRESS REPORT

Week ending: _____

	This Week	Month-to-Date
A. Total Charges posted	$	$
B. Total write-offs/ adjustments	$	$
C. Total receipts posted	$	$
D. A/R balance	$	$
	(End of this week)	(End of last week)

A/R ratios

    A/R to charges: (D÷A) = _____

                                                 (Last week)

    A/R to receipts: (D÷C) = _____

                                                 (Last week)

Number of patients

Total number of
rejected claims

Number of statements mailed

Mail returns

Comments:

CHAPTER 3

IDENTIFYING AND OVERSEEING VARIOUS FINANCIAL CLASSES

It is normal procedure for a practice to send monthly bills to patients who owe it money. A statement is sent to each individual and is usually typewritten or computer generated, although it can be a photostat of the patient's ledger. Some large practices with more advanced systems produce statements automatically and eliminate balances which are too low, flagging them for write-off. That's what normally happens. However, sending a monthly statement to some patients can be a waste of time, while for other patients a monthly statement may not be enough. Receivables are essentially locked into categories in regard to how they will eventually be paid; we refer to these categories as financial classes or payer classes, and each should be handled in a different manner to be the most effective.

Financial Classification Determines Future Action

To properly classify accounts by financial class, it is important to have as much correct information as possible about your patients. Classification by financial class will ultimately determine a number of things, such as the length of billing cycle, messages on statements, and other types of follow-up, such as which tools are best suited for achieving timely and efficient recovery of a receivable. For example, for patients classified as self-pay with no indication of any type of third party coverage, an immediate appeal for the use of MasterCard or Visa is appropriate. Obviously, that type of appeal will be ineffective with a patient who is covered under a group insurance plan. In this case, follow-up phone calls to the insurance company or a form letter to the state insurance commissioner may be the correct follow-up procedure.

In addition, when the patient is accurately classified by financial class, certain assumptions can be made about what's going to happen with that receivable. A practice may assume that all accounts receivable will be paid within 90 days and begin monitoring accounts only after receivables reach 90 days of age. However, there are some financial classes that should be expected to be paid in 30 days or less, while for some classes payment should be expected to take several months. Keep in mind that a charge for a self-pay patient is technically due at the time of service, not 30 days later. In theory, a self-pay account that gets to 30 days of age should be considered delinquent. Allowing those patients an extra 60 days before monitoring begins is a mistake because whatever reason a patient had for not paying in 30 days or less can be greater at the end of 90 days. The longer the problem goes unchallenged, the harder it is to collect the account.

Other financial classes may have a payment track of 120 days, and monitoring them at 90 days would be a waste of effort. For example, if you signed a contract for managed care which specifies that payment will be made within 120 days, it does little good to start pursuing payment of those charges before 120 days. If part of your practice involves Medicaid, which in your locale has a historical payment pattern of 150 days, you are spinning your wheels in trying to do something at 90 days. Each financial class has a historical perspective that is based on geographic location and discipline. It is important for a practice to tailor follow-up procedures to those norms, recognizing that some financial classes need immediate follow-up and others can wait.

Watch For Red Flags

Although it is important to gather correction information at the beginning, be aware that certain elements of information suggest a future collection problem, even before the account becomes a receivable. We call these warning signs "red flags." They are universal indicators of problems yet to come. Following are some examples of red flags to watch for:

Patient with a Rural Route for a Home Address

I worked as a bill collector my senior year in college in Johnson County, Indiana. I had been raised in a metropolitan area where everyone had a street address. As a collector, I had a difficult time adjusting to the system of mail delivery by rural route. A rural route can run 30 miles or more, and as I quickly learned, a rural route number was not a great indicator of where an individual lived. Therefore, when we received an account for collection with a rural route number, it raised a red flag, and we knew it might be difficult to find the exact location of the debtor because we often did knock on doors in our pursuit of debtors. Although a rural route address does not normally indicate a problem, extra time and effort should be made to obtain home and work phone numbers as a precaution.

Post Office Box as Patient's Home Address

A red flag should automatically pop up when a patient gives a post office box as his or her home address. A post office box can become a brick wall when one is trying to collect an account after a patient has been treated and is gone. Of course, there are genuine reasons for having a post office box. For example, in a metropolitan environment, particularly in a high-rise apartment building, a resident will often have mail delivered incorrectly because of the number of boxes in the lobby. That individual may choose to rent a post office box to assure timely and accurate delivery of mail. Also, a consumer may feel insecure about the mail delivery system and prefer to have mail locked at a more secure location, such as the post office. However, a post office box also can suggest a transient or unstable person. There may be problems trying to collect from this type of person down the line. Therefore, although a post office box can be a legitimate mailing address, obtaining the actual place of residence is critical for good A/R management.

No Home Phone Number

The patient who cannot provide a residential phone number can represent a collection problem yet to come. This poses a problem for the practice if the patient needs to be recalled. When a patient does not have a home phone, extra effort should be made to understand how phone communication can be made with patient now and in the future. An immediate family member, a close neighbor, and a work phone are second-best substitutes if the patient really does not have a home phone.

In Care Of

The patient who tells you to send the bill in care of another person or place usually has a much bigger story to tell. "In care of" can mean a temporary residence. Although there are many legitimate reasons why a patient's mail should be addressed in care of someone else, due diligence should be given to learning how to reach this patient if he or she leaves the current location. For example, our company acquired a batch of new accounts that had been given to us for collection. They appeared to include a reasonably high percentage of patients whose addresses were in care of someone else. The provider of services could be classified as an immediate care practice, and we spent a lot of time trying to understand why there were so many of these cases. It turned out that 80 percent of those addresses were for individuals from foreign countries who were traveling in the United States and had become ill during their stay. A large percentage were on some type of exchange program, and the residents at the addresses where they had stayed had little knowledge of their addresses in their countries of origin and certainly felt no responsibility.

A small percentage of these accounts, less than 5 percent, represented individuals who were in transit, staying with a relative. Normally they were staying because of a depressed financial situation and the relative had no desire to be of assistance in providing an address to which the patient had moved. As demonstrated in both cases, having a patient's address in care of another person can affect the eventual collectibility of the receivable. Although in many cases there is a legitimate explanation, alternate addresses should be obtained if possible.

Guarantor's Surname Different From Patient's Surname

A red flag should go up when a patient's last name is different from the guarantor's. Although this can be a common occurrence, there should be some explanation of their relationship. If care is not taken to get an explanation, the guarantor may tell you at a later date that he or she has no responsibility for the bill because he or she only transported the patient to the place of service. A common scenario goes like this: A patient requires immediate medical care, and the individual the patient had been living with takes her to the local hospital. During registration, the guarantor gives his or her name, which is of course different from the patient's name. The patient is discharged from the hospital, and some form of payment plan is arranged. However, soon after discharge, the patient decides to moves. The person the patient was living with now receives running notices since he or she was picked up as a guarantor and denies any liability for the medical treatment. Moreover, the guarantor has no idea where the patient is. Somewhere along the line someone should have questioned the different names and asked for additional information relative to the patient, not the guarantor. Open discussion in cases like this can often dispel misunderstanding at a later date.

Missing Zip Code

A completed patient information card that is missing the zip code may be more than a sign of absentmindedness. It can suggest transient behavior and a lack of permanency. You may find a zip code map of your area to be an extremely beneficial aide, particularly if you are in a metropolitan area where the same street names run through four or five communities. By quickly matching the zip code with the community and the patient information card, you may reduce the number of mail returns from the start.

Red Flags for Hospital-Based Practices

For practices that are primarily hospital-based and get patient information from hospital records, this challenge can be exasperating. Take the case of a hospital located within three blocks of a major county jail and one block of a major rehabilitation center. The hospital has an agreement with both facilities to treat their inmates and rehab patients. As these patients are brought to the hospital, invariably the address captured is that of the facility, which is usually not a permanent address. Nevertheless, the information is filtered out to the ancillary physicians. In this scenario, those responsible for inputting should become aware of red flag addresses whether they are transient hotels, halfway houses, rehab institutes or no address at all.

Financial Classes Of Payers

An A/R should be broken down into financial classes for the most effective management. The most prominent and common financial classes are self-pay, commercial insurance, workmen's compensation, managed or contractual care, Medicare, public aid or Medicaid, accident claims or claims with an attorney, and capitative care.

Self-Pay

A patient under the category of self-pay has no insurance or the policy of the practice is not to accept assignment of insurance. These patients are required to pay at the time of service. Self-pay also refers to the portion of a bill that is not covered by insurance or any other type of third party payment, which would include the patient's deductible and co-payment portions. This payer class undoubtedly ranks as the number one challenge in controlling A/R and should constitute the smallest percentage of any given financial class. Unpaid self-pays older than 30 days can become collection problems.

As a result, self-pay should have the shortest billing cycle, and a concentrated effort to get the best demographic information and collection effort at the time of service is essential. However, a large percentage of the disciplines in healthcare have little control over this. Hospital-based practices such as anesthesiology, radiology, and pathology more often than not have no alternative and must treat all patients. Nevertheless, regardless of discipline, when a patient is classified as self-pay, it is imperative to identify that patient as soon as possible for the quickest action. For example, the charges for an individual coming through the emergency room with demographic information that suggest he or she lives on the street should be disposed as quickly as possible. If you recognize that in all probability collection is impossible, it is much more efficient and economical to write-off a receivable on the day of service than to let it bog down the system. In most practices, patients who have balances after third party insurance are changed to a self-pay status. For tracking purposes, it may be a good policy to have two self-pay classifications: original bill and balance after insurance.

Because you are a business, consideration should be given to a number of alternatives that you are willing to offer your self-pay patients to get them to pay at the time of service. The use of major credit cards such as MasterCard, Visa and American Express is one alternatives. Although the discount rate the bank charges for this service varies, it may strike you as being expensive at first glance. For example, if your average charge is $80 and the discount rate is 3 or 4 percent, the thought of spending $2.40 to $3.20 to have the bill paid at the time of service may not seem attractive. In all probability, however, when you consider the cost of generating the first statement, the probability of having to send several statements, and the risk of the account going delinquent, you will quickly realize that fee is more than justified. Also, offering the use of a credit card for payment, becomes a backup support for your staff and sends a message to your patients, particularly if you are trying to collect from all patients at the time of service. It gives your staff another response to the patient who says "I forgot my checkbook," and helps reinforce to the patient that you are serious about the policy. However, the use of a credit card will be attractive and effective for only a limited number of your patients, especially those in the self-pay classification.

Commercial Insurance

This classification is traditionally used for patients who still have coverage under the traditional third party coverage system, whether through their employers or as private insurance. In many areas of the country this type of coverage is shrinking dramatically because of the presence of a host of managed healthcare contracts. Two of the most common problems in collecting assigned benefits from these companies are incorrect policy numbers and the lack of a mailing address for a claim. It is a classification, along with Medicare, that should have the shortest time cycle for payment and the highest level of reimbursement. In essence, if you're a/R is categorized by financial class and you have many claims of this type going beyond 30 days, you should be concerned.

Inherent in this classification, however, is a problem that grows daily: the concept of the usual and customary charge. For years, the patient was treated and an insurance form was submitted to the carrier. Payment was received in a reasonable time frame, usually for 80 percent or more of the bill. However, that scenario has changed dramatically. Now the payment invariably is accompanied by a letter to the subscriber stating that the bill the insurance company has received is over the limits of usual and customary charges and as a result, the insurance company will not make the expected payment. If it knows in advance that this can be a problem, the practice can reduce it by having the patient sign an agreement that he or she is responsible for the entire bill regardless of what the insurance pays or allows. This won't solve every problem, but it may remind the patient that you did not participate in the selection of insurance and that this is strictly an issue between the patient and their insurance company. Further discussion of policy regarding usual and customary charges is included in Chapter 5.

Worker's Compensation

No patient should be place into this payer class unless there is written authorization from the employer that this is indeed a work-related injury or phone verification that this should be treated as a worker's compensation case. With the high cost of worker's compensation in most states today, more compensation cases are being contested.

Therefore, any statement by the employer that an injury is work related will reduce the probability that four to six months after the time of service you will find yourself billing the group insurance rather than the compensation carrier. This not only inflates you're a/R, but may be rejected by the group insurance because of late filing.

Managed Care or Contractual Care

Regardless of the combination of alphabetical letters managed care coverage comes under—HMO (health maintenance organization), PPO (preferred provider organization), or IPA (independent practice association)—the receivable needs to be managed just as the care was. Since in many cases there will be some form of contractual relationship between a managed care company and your practice, and since these contracts can vary dramatically, it is best for monitoring purposes to have this type of payer class broken out under each of the individual contracts. All too often a physician signs a contract with a high discount rate that is based on payment within 30 days. If the receivable gets lumped with all other managed healthcare receivables, there is no way to track whether the 30-day commitment is being kept.

This is also an area where the entire staff has to be familiar with the commitments the practice has made as well as those the practice did not make. The problems of pre-authorization, along with slow pay and variations of copay, make this a very challenging category to oversee. In some extreme cases, managed care contracts have been known to bring a practice to bankruptcy. Suppose a practice commits itself contractually to a small neighborhood managed care group. The contract contains no provisions about what will happen if that organization merges with a larger network. Shortly after the contract is signed, that is precisely what occurs. Suddenly the practice is faced with the fact that it entered a relationship which it perceived would account for no more than a small percentage of its total patients and is now inundated to a point where the actual proportion of patients seen under the contractual agreement approaches 50 percent, all at a high discount rate.

Imagine a practice that has entered into several agreements, all with different protocols for treatment, reimbursement levels and settlement schedules. All of this is done without any guarantee from the managed care unit that it will furnish various forms of provider support, such as a monthly report on the status of the claims. As a result, the practice quickly realizes that to stay on top, it is going to have to add one or more full-time employees to make sure the contract is functioning as stated in the agreement. There may not be any provisions or remedies for situations where the contract is not functioning as it should.

Then there is the case where a hospital enters into a contractual relationship and not all physician members have joined. Even if a practice has no direct relationship with the managed care group, this can make public relations and collections difficult. We hear more and more of the following type of response: "I specifically went to that hospital because they were part of my PPO, and I thought all the charges would be covered. How was I to know that some of the physicians at the hospital were not members?"

It is important to remember that there is a triangular involvement in managed care: physician, managed care organization, and patient. Envision the following scenario: In a very large metropolitan community there is a large HMO with high name recognition. In reality, the HMO consists of 92 individual and separate sites, each one self-administered. A patient joining this HMO is registered at one of the sites, but because of the name identification, he perceives that he is part of the entire network. It is determined that his spouse needs some extremely specialized care. There is a site within the HMO that has a physician with a specialty in the type of care needed. The patient is therefore removed from the registration list of the first site and moved to the other site, but new identification cards are not issued. However, at the new site the primary physician who will be treating the patient is aware of what's taking place. The patient is admitted, and has extensive surgery, but the insurance card given at the time of admission shows the old site. Those practitioners and the hospital that verified coverage before service was rendered received a positive response. Since it took more than 90 days to remove the patient from the first site, that site is billed and in due time, the bills are rejected. After more than 90 days it is discovered what has occurred, and the appropriate site is billed. However, the resubmitted claims are rejected because more than 90 days has elapsed from the time of service, which is one of the provisions of the contract. In the worst-case scenario this occurs in one of three states that have special HMO protection (Illinois, Maryland and Florida) so that the patient can't be pursued for payment.

Although this doesn't occur every day, it can and does happen. Many specialty societies in organized healthcare have prepared information handouts on what a given specialty should look for in a managed care contract or even a capitation care contract. It may be advisable for a practice to inquire whether information for its discipline is available.

Medicare

Assuming that you are a participating physician in the Medicare program, this financial payer class should be one of the easiest to manage, provided that you have the capacity to submit electronic media claims (EMC) and immediately move the patient's copay status to self-pay upon receiving payment from Medicare. In most areas of the country Medicare payment is made within 21 days for EMCs. Therefore, if your billing is timely, the number of Medicare receivables that age beyond 30 days should be extremely small and any Medicare account still open at 90 days should be clearly identified as a problem.

Although EMC is mentioned here for this payer class, it obviously affects many other financial classes, particularly commercial insurance. Healthcare administration is moving toward a paperless environment. Although the concept of electronically submitted claims is not new, many practices still do not use this technology. This topic is discussed in greater depth in Chapter 11, and its importance cannot be overemphasized. Medicare intermediaries are under a mandate to increase the level of participation by physicians for EMC, and as time passes, practices that have not moved into this arena will find it more difficult to manage their receivables. Right now the payment floor of 21 days for EMC as opposed to 45 days for paper claims represents a significant penalty. More importantly, the more aggressive practices in this area have already moved on to electronic remittances. The electronic data highway will be a significant factor in the efficient management of receivables.

Public Aid/Medicaid

The problems inherent in this financial class vary from state to state. However, if you were able to get the correct demographic information at the very beginning, this class should be reasonably manageable because there is no interface with the patient. However, if you are consistently involved in obtaining information from the patient to get a claim paid, or if your practice has a high percentage of Medicaid patients, you should explore the technology that is involved in your state. For example, for a monthly charge, some states allow for a modem link directly to the physician's practice to verify public aid eligibility for each service date. If that is not available or if the volume of the practice is too small to justify the cost, a photostat of the Medicaid card is mandatory, making sure the card reflects the coverage dates for treatment. A card for the month before the date of service is no guarantee that the patient is eligible. Another consideration is that in many states the Medicaid budget runs out prior to the end of the fiscal year. Therefore, it is not uncommon to see lapses of payments of several weeks to several months. This is important if a high percentage of your patient care involves Medicaid. Additional cash flow planning is necessary.

Accident Claims or Claims with an Attorney

This financial class normally represents patients who were treated by you for some form of injury for which litigation is taking place. In most practices this is an extremely small category, and if its done correctly in the beginning, it requires little management. This includes taking the time to file a physician's lien on all concerns parties. A physician's lien is a legal document that varies from state to state but clearly specifies that you rendered medical services for the treatment of injuries sustained by the injured party; the lien also states the name of the person allegedly liable for payment. Normally, this notice is served both to the injured party and to the person or persons allegedly liable. It is best to consult an attorney about the type of physician's lien required in your area.

Although not foolproof, the physician's lien helps ensure that you get some portion of the settlement when the case is finally heard. Periodic letters to the attorney asking about the status also helps control this financial class. However, keep in mind that a patient may be placed in this classification even though benefits are available through the patient's group insurance.

Capitative Care

Capitation is a method of payment for health services in which an individual or institutional provider is paid a fixed per-capita amount for each person served without regard to the number or nature of services provided. Capitative care differs from managed care in that under the capitation method the physician bears the risk whereas under the most common concepts of managed care, he or she simply takes a discount. It is also important to remember that there can be modifiers in the more sophisticated capitation care agreements. The actuaries who design these agreements use terms such as "threshold," which represents the limit of service that will be rendered under the capitative method. Once that level of care is reached, there should be some form of reevaluation. Another term used in capitative care agreements is "carve-outs," referring to procedures which are uncommon or unusually high in cost and are not considered part of the capitation care for that population.

As capitative care becomes more common it needs to be given consideration for the purposes of computer planning. The way most computer programs are designed, a patient master is set up, and as charges are incurred, they are posted to that patient. This in turn generates a billing statement to a third party payer, the patient, or both. Envision the technology that would be necessary to accept a roster of 10,000 patients, along with the quarterly lump sum payment. It is still necessary to track the amount of care rendered to individuals in this population and monitor when a threshold is met on each one individually. Moreover, there will have to be provisions for the carve-outs so that they are not considered part of the capitation. Finally, rather than generating billing statements, the system will generate sophisticated management reports which will have to be monitored with a great deal of intensity to make sure you haven't sold your practice short.

Timeline For Resolution By Financial Class

Each financial class has its own timeline for resolution. Treating these classes separately will create savings in postage costs and frustration as well as provide the ability to monitor them for better control of A/R. More important, handling them independently will give a more accurate view of the practice's accounts receivable. Realistically, a practice needs a timeline matrix for billing and collection for each financial class. For example, a monthly statement is automatically sent to each patient for a period of five months before an account becomes delinquent and other steps such as collection are considered. That's wrong. A once-a-month billing cycle for five months may be alright for some of your financial classes, but it is too long for some and perhaps much too short for others.

Another reason to deal with A/R by financial class is accuracy in the prediction of income for planning purposes. One can't simply look at an A/R and use the historical performance for that area to make a determination that a certain percentage will be collected. There can be trouble down the road if one does not look at each financial class individually. Each of these financial classes has a different value as a percentage of recovery. If a practice has a high number of self-pays, the calculations can be wrong by 50% or more. Therefore, the ability to view A/R by financial class is critical, as is the capacity to tailor billing cycles and messages on statements. If you modify billing cycles and alter the messages on statements, a more realistic expectation level will be achieved and the use of personnel time for efforts that are nonproductive will be avoided.

Knowing what to expect from each financial class will help in modifying your billing procedures. Listed below are examples of what you can reasonably expect from several financial classes in regard to billing cycles.

Self-Pay

As mentioned previously, in the case of self-pay, the day the charge for services rendered to the patient was entered into the system is the day the receivable is due. In reality, the charge becomes delinquent on the second day; more realistically it is considered past due at 30 days. Assuming that the matrix of the overall billing cycle is 150 days, why wait an additional 120 days before taking more aggressive steps? In other words, why give self-pay patients the same course of action as the other financial classes?

A policy towards self-pays may include a provision that a patient is contacted within several days of the initial billing. Better yet, mandate that the patient is contacted even before the initial billing to ascertain that he or she is indeed self-pay and at the same time, establish the manner in which the bill will be resolved. Again, it is important that your staff have many alternatives available, such as the use of MasterCard and Visa, and guidelines for acceptable payment plans. In many cases, simply giving a staff member the authority to move an account immediately to collection may be a good alternative. Although a similar concept is necessary for each financial class, the one entitled self-pay can't wait.

Medicare Claims

As stated earlier, Medicare claims that are submitted electronically should be paid within 30 days or less. For Medicare patients with copayment due, the patient's portion should be expected at the end of 30 days and treated as a self-pay at that time. Any assigned Medicare account that is not under review and that is 45 to 60 days of age or one with no personal payment activity or patient communication should be considered delinquent. Therefore, at 90 days any additional statements cost you money and valuable time in the majority of cases.

Managed Care Claims

The length of time a managed care claim should be in your billing cycle is dependent on the contractual arrangement that was made with the managed care organization. For example, if a contract stated that an HMO has 120 days to make the payment, technically one would be spinning one's wheels by doing anything but wait until then. However, some steps should be taken to assure prompt payment by the 120th day. The most important step is to develop a method by which the managed care organization acknowledges the receipt of a claim. With that in place, at the end of 4 months the HMO cannot say that it never received a claim in the first place. Also, even though a contract may give the HMO 120 days to make payment, realistically it should be made in a much shorter period of time, particularly if a discount is involved. Therefore, ideally, an arrangement is made by which the managed care organization agrees to acknowledge by fax, phone, or some other method all claims that have been submitted, including claims that have been submitted in batches. Then, at the end of 30 days, one should take any steps that are available, such as canceling the discount.

Commercial Insurance

The timelines for insurance claims vary greatly depending on the type of insurance and whether an electronic clearinghouse is being used for claims. Larger carriers usually will be able to say what their average turnaround time is. Whether that is acceptable is beyond your control, but at least it can be a guideline so that steps can be taken for follow-up if the claim is not paid within that period.

Realistic Billing Cycle

Aside from special cases such as Medicare assignments, managed care cases, and public aid claims, here are various timelines and options for realistic billing cycles.

Day of Service

If a patient was physically seen in the office, you have several options on the day of service. You can do the following:

1. Ask the patient to pay and collect at the time of service.

2. Get insurance information from the patient and submit a claim to the carrier.

3. Require the patient to pay for that amount which will not be covered by insurance and/or Medicare.

4. Give the patient a detailed "superbill," collect the payment, and leave the responsibility for insurance reimbursement to the patient.

In cases where a patient was not physically seen in the office, such as in surgery or hospital care, and in cases where the patient did not pay at the time of service, the patient must be billed. Here are some timelines for action.

Billing Action I: Send Bill to Patient on Day of Service

The best method is to send a bill to the patient on the day of service or as soon afterward as possible. This is true for all financial classes except those in which the patient has no responsibility, such as contractual care and public aid. When a claim has been filed with the patient's insurance provider, it informs the patient of his or her liability. However, why waste postage? Send a statement after the insurance has paid its portion.

Take this one step further and envision a worker's compensation claim. There is a definite benefit in forming the patient that there is a financial liability if the claim is protested and not paid by the carrier. The same is true in sending a statement to a patient who has third party coverage. Not only is the patient notified of the financial obligation, but he or she also can change any information that is incorrect. A further benefit of billing all patients right away is that it will draw out incorrect addresses in the form of a mail return which will be relatively easy to correct very early in the billing cycle. Finally, if a patient has any complaints about the care rendered or amount the charged, it is far easier to deal with the problems immediately after you provide the care.

Billing Action II: At 30 Days

If payment has not been received by the end of 30 days, a patient is billed again. In cases of insurance assignments, a statement is sent asking the patient to contact the insurance company about the delay or a statement is sent telling the patient that the charge is his or her responsibility. However, not everyone needs a bill every 30 days, as in the financial classes of public aid and worker's compensation. If self-pay patients are not contacted within the first five days after service, asking them how the bill should be handled, they certainly should be contacted by the end of 30 days. Again, if you sort an A/R by financial class, the proper steps can be taken to ensure the best outcome.

Billing Action III: At 60 Days

At the end of 60 days, with receivables sorted by financial class, one should have a realistic view of what can be expected. You should know who should be paying and what may be delaying the payment. At this point it is time to work accounts with the highest return first. In other words, begin taking action on the financial class that has the highest known rate of recovery. It is also best to work accounts with the largest balances first. Separate those classes over which there is no control from the normal billing cycle, such as managed care and public aid claims, and put them in abeyance until they become delinquent.

If you recognize the highest-risk accounts and treat them aggressively early on, you will allow your staff members to focus on what is truly collectible. If a practice has a large volume of unpaid self-pays at the end of 60 days, it is wise to outsource those accounts so that a concentrated effort can be made to get them paid or to obtain information that may help settle them in another way. My company provides this service to a major teaching department at a hospital, and we normally get 35 percent of self-pay accounts reclassified as either Medicaid or legal status. If the department had waited longer, very often these patients would have been hard to contact or would have moved.

Change Billing Strategy

It may be necessary to change your billing strategy in order to achieve the best results in managing A/R. As consumers, most people acknowledge who they owe and why. That is not always true of ancillary services in healthcare. For example, how many patients are surprised and angry when they receive a bill for ECG interpretation? Many have no recollection nor do not feel an obligation to the physician. Recognize the fact that when you are granting credit, a simple assumption is made that the patient acknowledges the obligation to you and really want to pay. There is even an attitude among some people that, "Yes, I know I owe, but I'm not going to pay. They're rich.

They don't need my money." In some cases it is time to adopt a new billing strategy and change the routine and your manner for approaching the situation to get good results.

Billing Options

Most physician billing offices try to mail a statement of the indebtedness to the responsible party between the 28th of the month and the 5th of the following month, with the belief that the debtor receives most of his bills toward the first of each month so your bill should be right there, too. There are four billing options here.

Option 1: Send a single bill to all patients once a month, at the same time each month.

The net effect of this type of billing is that a tremendous amount of additional work is required to get a once-a-month bill out, followed by an influx of payments and phone calls shortly thereafter, creating peaks and valleys of cash flow and work flow. Also, during the billing process, even if a staff member notices a statement going to a patient when something else should happen, because of time pressure, there isn't a chance to deal with it.

Option 2: Send bills to patients twice a month.

Divide the alphabet in half and bill all patients with a last name beginning with A to M on the 15th of the month and all patients with a last name beginning with N to Z on the 31st. Although this will help reduce the large hump in workload that occurs with monthly billing, a two-hump system has been created with a double peak and valley effect. To some degree this is even more unfavorable since the humps are still large enough to be troublesome and rather than being distracted once a month, you are doing it twice.

Option 3: Bill one-fourth of the accounts each week.

This weekly cycle billing is a vast improvement over options 1 and 2, but depending on the size of the practice, it is not the most effective type of cycle billing.

Option 4: Send bills to patients on the anniversary of the initial service date.

This is the ultimate billing procedure. In theory, approximately 1/28 of all patients will receive a bill every day, distributing the workload over the entire month, along with the incoming phone calls, cash posting, and follow-up of insurance.

Change to Cycle Billing

One of the largest department stores in the United States found that rather than doing weekly cycle billing, it was better to bill the accounts alphabetically, such as A on the first, B on the second, and so on. By doing this, they found that they could distribute the cash flow without reducing collections. Therefore, it is recommended that monthly statements be billed in some form of cycle, preferably daily, to distribute the workload. Moreover, with cycle billing the income becomes more dispersed, as do the complaints and incoming phone calls, so that staff members won't view the five days after a massive billing as a disaster. In fact, the postage costs, the return mail, and all other work-related procedures tied into billing will be spread more evenly over a 30-day period, avoiding the peak-and-valley effect. Distributing your billing cycle over a full month may be advantageous not only to your economic health, but to the well-being of your employees.

Vary the Size and Type of Envelope

Every month a statement is mailed with the same type of envelope to all the patients owe money. In some cases a message is printed on the statement that shows an increasing dismay at the lack of payment. Let's take a moment and think about that. People who don't plan to pay or can't pay won't even open the envelope to read the message. They know what's in the envelope and will toss it aside.

For the sake of diversity and to grab attention, consider adopting different sizes or types of envelopes at critical points in the billing cycle, ones with which the patient won't be so familiar. At 60 days of age the statements could be mailed in number 10 envelopes with the return address on the back, rather than in the usual smaller window envelope with the return address on the front. You are trying to get the patient's attention and get a response. Although many companies provide precollect services that do just that, much can be achieved simply by altering the type of envelope you use.

The Use of Color in Billing

There is another consideration in calling attention to the monthly statement. Colors are an extremely effective psychological method that are used infrequently because of the cost of inventory. However, as a challenge, try mailing 60- or 90-day notices in a bright pink envelope or loud yellow envelope, and I believe you will notice a significant increase in the response rate. Another possibility is to use a bright pink return envelope for the patient to mail back his or her payment. This would be an added benefit because as the postal carrier brings the mail, your staff members will know if they have gotten through to the patient. Although many professionals do not consider this an option, many offices already send the final notice in a similar way, with a big red stamp that says "If Not Paid in 10 Days This Account Will Be Referred to Collection." Expand the concept early in the process. Remember that you are in competition with many other credit granters. Some may even be your peers or work at the hospital where you practice. You are in competition, and if you are going to control you're a/R, you need to consider alternatives. Color can be effective.

Other Attention-Getters

There are other ways to get the attention of a party that owes you money. Here are some hints that may help in this process. Although they may not be cost-efficient, they are known to work.

1. The typical consumer almost always opens first the mail that has stamps and may ignore letters that have imprints from a mail machine. A postage stamp infers something personal and therefore perhaps friendly and gets first attention.

2. The typical consumer also opens hand-addressed envelopes before machine-addressed envelopes or one with labels, especially if he doesn't know where it is coming from.

The ultimate attention grabber would be a bright yellow number 10 envelope hand addressed with a postage stamp. It should certainly get the attention and response for which you are looking, although it may not be cost-feasible because of the time it takes your staff to produce it. I know of one case where an envelope was designed so that it didn't quite meet at the seal and revealed part of the contents of the envelope. It was hand addressed and had a return address created by a massive rubber stamp which said "RECEIVABLE DEPARTMENT—XYZ CLINIC." You could see a pink return envelope through the cracks in the outgoing envelope, and the outside envelope had a colorful postage stamp. You can bet it got opened first. Again, you have to alter your style to get the patient's attention, and being creative can be an advantage.

Messages Within The Statement

Most practices and billing companies spend a great deal of time and effort deciding what type of insert and message a statement should carry. Several companies have made untold dollars selling to medical practices and facilities "proven and effective messages" to put on billing statements. On deeper examination, it is often noted that they have used some of the techniques we mentioned earlier, such as bright colors and a different type of envelope. In effect, what the message says is not necessarily what triggers the response.

There are some things to remember in designing the wording for a statement. What you are trying to do is to persuade the patient to pay. For the most part, the recipient understands what is wanted. The fact that there was a request for money is what usually creates the response, not so much what is said. However, in the belief that the message on the statement is important to you and the patient, remember these points:

1. Messages should be short. A long and wordy message probably will not be read.

2. The message should be in simple language, straight and to the point. Even picture stories have been shown to be effective. Medicare started using child-like stick figures of patients going to the mailbox to explain that when the form was completed, it should be mailed to Medicare.

3. Consider translations into other languages, such as Spanish, depending on the location of your practice. This is a major consideration that is based on the ability of your staff, but remember that patients are looking for reasons *not* to pay you. Is a language barrier one of them?

4. Messages should not be redundant. A final notice that is sent more than once has truly lost its impact and can limit what you or a collection agency can do. It is like telling employees that they can't be late to work more than four times. At the fifth tardiness, you tell them they have one more chance. When do you really mean it?

5. Make it clear what is expected and what action will be taken. Discontinuing service to a patient may seem overkill, but one needs to decide what that delinquency means to the entire office.

The Personal Collection Letter

After you have used colored envelopes with concise messages explaining exactly what is expected and a self-pay patient has not responded to your statements, it is good practice to send that patient a personal collection letter before making any phone calls. It should be personally addressed to the patient or the responsible party and typed on letterhead paper so that it does not look like a form letter with the blanks filled in. With sophisticated word processing and personal computers, it is relatively simple to make each letter look as though it was written directly to an individual.

Make it Short and To The Point

The letter should not be too lengthy. Studies show that the probability of readership of a letter declines as the number of words increases. A collection letter of 40 words or less will be read by close to 100 percent of the people while a letter of 150 words or more will be read by only 50 percent. The letter should be clearly stated, using simple and direct words. Sometimes underlining or highlighting important words calls attention to them.

Carefully Select the Words You Use

Your letter should convey the feeling that you are trying to help the patient as well as preserve his dignity and self respect. The words and phrases you use should be positive and optimistic, such as "your cooperation," "successful conclusion," "mutual satisfaction," "assurance," "conviction," and "advantageous." Avoid the use of antagonizing words and phrases such as "insist," "demand," "failure," "delinquent," "you allege," "you claim," "you said you would," "deficiency," and "displeased." A good collection letter should end with a compelling request: "I expect your payment of $85 in full by Friday at noon. Please call my office by noon Friday if you find this to be impossible."

Appeal to Their Emotions

Your ultimate goal is to give the patient an opportunity to voluntarily pay the bill. This is done by arousing their emotions of pride, honesty, self-interest, and fear.

Encourage a Sense of Pride

Stress the importance of good citizenship and reputation in the community. Honorable and respectful men and women pay their bills promptly. Some examples include: *"You're a hard-working individual. I am sure you wouldn't want anything like this to jeopardize your good standing." "Isn't your good reputation worth more than $__?"*

Appeal to Feelings of Honesty

Appeal to the patient's honesty and sense of fair play. You rendered services to the patient with complete confidence that he or she intended to pay the bill. Try writing, *"I know you want to be paid for the work that you do. In all fairness, we rendered a service to you when you needed it. Now it is your turn to pay." "Don't you think it is only fair to do the right thing and pay the balance in full?"*

Appeal to Self-Interest

Appeal to the patient's own self-interest by stressing the importance of paying the balance in full to preserve his or her credit rating, avoid additional expenses, and maintain peace of mind. *"Aren't you concerned about your family's credit rating? You owe it to them to pay in full now." "If you pay now, you'll avoid additional expenses for interest and rebilling fees later on." "Preserve the financial security of your family. Pay the balance today."*

Appeal to Fear

Although you don't want to overdo this type of appeal, it is usually the last step and usually includes a warning that the account is going to be referred to a collection agency unless it is paid in full. *"It is unfortunate that you are willing to ruin your good credit rating for $___. The collection agency we use always reports debts to the credit bureau." "If we do not receive payment by the end of the month, we will refer this account to our collection agency. It will be extremely inconvenient for you if you need to apply for credit in the future."*

After you send the personalized collection letter and there has been no response within a reasonable period of time, say two or three weeks, it is time to make a collection phone call. This will be fully discussed in Chapter 7.

Summary

Each financial class in a practice has a certain distinct paying habit which should be identified. These financial classes include self-pay, commercial insurance, Medicare, public aid, managed care, worker's compensation, attorney cases, and capitative care. If possible, each financial class should be treated differently in the management of A/R. It is important to obtain correct information so that you can properly categorize each patient and heed red flags such as a post office box as a home address, a patient wanting to be billed in care of someone else, and a guarantor whose last name is different from the patient. These situations may cause problems in collection at a later date.

Each financial class has its own timeline for resolution. A self-pay account is due at the time of service, while payment under a managed care contract is due in accordance with the terms of the contract. Bills generally are sent to patients once a month, but by changing billing strategy, for example with cycle billing, you can obtain better results in controlling A/R. Be creative in the use of color, size, and type of envelope, and make sure the messages on statements are concise and to the point. If a patient has not responded within a reasonable time frame, before making collection calls send a personal collection letter. Make it short and to the point, and appeal to the emotions of the patient by encouraging the sense of pride, and feelings of honesty, self-interest and fear.

The real success comes from recognizing the differences in the financial classes. But more important is not holding accounts for extended periods. If they have gone through your treatment process without result, get rid of them. They will cost you more than you recover using internal resources. There is one constant to everything I have seen in medical A/R management and that is every practice that holds accounts beyond their billing cycle has one or more problems with their A/R.

CHAPTER 4

BILLING SYSTEMS

A medical practice has a wide variety of choices in selecting a system that will manage receivables, produce statements for billing, and prepare insurance claim forms. Although some are dinosaurs, many of these systems are inexpensive and relatively uncomplicated. However, more practices, large and small, are equipping their offices with computers and software to manage their receivables. Whether a practice chooses a manual system or a computer program for billing and A/R management, each system has advantages and disadvantages. A quick look at these systems can be helpful.

Ledger Card

The ledger card is a simple one. Data regarding the patient, such as the patient's name, the responsible party's name, and sometimes a home phone number, are written onto a rigid rectangular card. Usually there is space to record charges, payments, the balance due, and dates of billing on the lower half of the card. Figure 4-1 shows a typical ledger card. The card is usually filed alphabetically and is pulled when a patient's medical file is retrieved for an office or hospital visit. Normally, a photostat made at the end of the month serves as the billing mechanism. This method is still used for billing patients in an economical and simple way.

The ledger card system has many disadvantages, however. Since CPT codes and ICD-9 codes usually are not shown on the ledger, it does not provide all the data needed for preparing CMS-1500 forms, those claim forms nearly all third party insurance carriers, including Medicare use. A sample CMS-1500 form is shown in Figure 4-2. Another disadvantage is that it cannot do much to control receivables. To obtain an aged A/R, the ledger cards have to be filed separately by age, creating a nightmare when trying to locate a patient's ledger. The greatest disadvantage occurs when try to tally a total A/R, monthly charges, or monthly payments. To do this, some form of subsystem and the use of an adding machine are required.

It is hard to use checks and balances with this system to ensure that all charges are posted. To obtain off-site backup for security reasons, an extra photostat of the ledger card has to be made monthly and stored off site, but this leaves the current month's work unprotected. It is a system highly prone to embezzlement, since there is little control over the

Figure 4-1: Sample ledger card

Robert M. Jones, M.D.
1234 Main Street
Hometown, IL 66006
(708) 123-4567

Mr. John R. Smith
4567 Elm Street
Hometown, IL 66006

For: Emily Smith   Phone: 555-3334

FOR PROFESSIONAL SERVICES
For Emily Smith

	Charge	Payment	Balance
Balance brought forward			$0
Initial office visit 1/2/03	$50.00	$50.00	0
Office visit 2/4/03	40.00		40.00
Injection 2/4/03	20.00		60.00
Statement sent 2/28/03			60.00
Office visit 3/8/03	40.00	100.00	0
Lab fees 3/9/03	22.00		22.00
Statement sent 3/30/03			22.00

individual A/R ledger cards. For a payment to disappear, the only requirement is that the ledger card also disappear. Even with its drawbacks, this system is inexpensive and easy to use.

Pegboard/One-Write Systems

The pegboard or one-write system is usually sold as a total manual system for controlling many aspects of the practice, including payables, check writing, patient charges, and payments. It is called a one-write system because every transaction in the office is recorded with one writing of a charge, a payment, or a payable through the use of carbon paper overlays on a pegboard, which holds everything in line. This system usually also includes a ledger card as the medium for posting charges and payments.

The pegboard system's main advantage over the ledger card is that it provides for numerous checks and balances and generates month-end reports. For example, when a check is written using various carbon overlays on a peg board, the germane information transferred to an accounts payable journal. In addition, when one uses carbon overlays to record a payment on the receipts ledger and on a patient's ledger card, all information is recorded in one transaction. These journals can be balanced daily with the receipts and charges of the day because they are physically all in one place. However, a payment on a ledger card system by itself does not tie back to the deposit that should have been made in the same time period. In other words, a pegboard system utilizes multiple recording of transactions, all of which are tied together, providing a paper trail of the transaction. By contract, a ledger card used as a stand alone makes paper trails of that nature virtually impossible.

The primary disadvantage of a pegboard is that is has to be manned by an individual at all times. It is not something that can be put aside and completed at the end of the day. Therefore, if the availability of personnel is uncertain, it could present a significant problem. On the positive side, it helps staff members request payment at time of service. Also, the method by which it is organized dictates that everything has to be entered on a carbon transfer form, which definitively helps keep everything organized and in one place. However, like the ledger card, it fails to allow the aging of receivables without extensive additional work. The ledger card and pegboard are examples of the technology of the 1940s to 1970s, but many practices still use them out of habit and because they are cost-efficient and relatively simple.

Super Bill

The late 1970's brought the concept of the superbill. Until that time, medical insurance as we know it today was a rarity. A new era of insurance companies, including Medicare, Blue Cross and Blue Shield, demanded accurate reporting of medical claims, including detailed information about the type of service and the diagnosis for which the service was rendered. As a result, practitioners had to scramble to find a method that would allow reporting of services rendered to a third party coverage without a lot of extra clerical help to complete insurance claim forms.

Normally, the super bill is a multipart form that contains preprinted information such as the name of the practitioner, tax ID numbers, and provider codes, along with blank space for the primary and secondary

Figure 4-2: A sample CMS-1500 form

PLEASE
DO NOT
STAPLE
IN THIS
AREA

APPROVED OMB-0938-0008

CARRIER

PICA

HEALTH INSURANCE CLAIM FORM

PICA

1. MEDICARE MEDICAID CHAMPUS CHAMPVA GROUP HEALTH PLAN FECA BLK LUNG OTHER   1a. INSURED'S I.D. NUMBER (FOR PROGRAM IN ITEM 1)

(Medicare #) (Medicaid #) (Sponsor's SSN) (VA File #) (SSN or ID) (SSN) (ID)

2. PATIENT'S NAME (Last Name, First Name, Middle Initial)

3. PATIENT'S BIRTH DATE   MM DD YY   SEX   M   F

4. INSURED'S NAME (Last Name, First Name, Middle Initial)

5. PATIENT'S ADDRESS (No., Street)

6. PATIENT RELATIONSHIP TO INSURED   Self   Spouse   Child   Other

7. INSURED'S ADDRESS (No., Street)

CITY   STATE

8. PATIENT STATUS   Single   Married   Other

CITY   STATE

ZIP CODE   TELEPHONE (Include Area Code) (   )

Employed   Full-Time Student   Part-Time Student

ZIP CODE   TELEPHONE (INCLUDE AREA CODE) (   )

9. OTHER INSURED'S NAME (Last Name, First Name, Middle Initial)

10. IS PATIENT'S CONDITION RELATED TO:

11. INSURED'S POLICY GROUP OR FECA NUMBER

a. OTHER INSURED'S POLICY OR GROUP NUMBER

a. EMPLOYMENT? (CURRENT OR PREVIOUS)   YES   NO

a. INSURED'S DATE OF BIRTH   MM DD YY   SEX   M   F

b. OTHER INSURED'S DATE OF BIRTH   MM DD YY   SEX   M   F

b. AUTO ACCIDENT?   YES   NO   PLACE (State)

b. EMPLOYER'S NAME OR SCHOOL NAME

c. EMPLOYER'S NAME OR SCHOOL NAME

c. OTHER ACCIDENT?   YES   NO

c. INSURANCE PLAN NAME OR PROGRAM NAME

d. INSURANCE PLAN NAME OR PROGRAM NAME

10d. RESERVED FOR LOCAL USE

d. IS THERE ANOTHER HEALTH BENEFIT PLAN?   YES   NO   *If yes,* return to and complete item 9 a-d.

READ BACK OF FORM BEFORE COMPLETING & SIGNING THIS FORM.
12. PATIENT'S OR AUTHORIZED PERSON'S SIGNATURE I authorize the release of any medical or other information necessary to process this claim. I also request payment of government benefits either to myself or to the party who accepts assignment below.

SIGNED   DATE

13. INSURED'S OR AUTHORIZED PERSON'S SIGNATURE I authorize payment of medical benefits to the undersigned physician or supplier for services described below.

SIGNED

14. DATE OF CURRENT: MM DD YY   ILLNESS (First symptom) OR INJURY (Accident) OR PREGNANCY(LMP)

15. IF PATIENT HAS HAD SAME OR SIMILAR ILLNESS. GIVE FIRST DATE   MM DD YY

16. DATES PATIENT UNABLE TO WORK IN CURRENT OCCUPATION   MM DD YY   FROM   TO   MM DD YY

17. NAME OF REFERRING PHYSICIAN OR OTHER SOURCE

17a. I.D. NUMBER OF REFERRING PHYSICIAN

18. HOSPITALIZATION DATES RELATED TO CURRENT SERVICES   MM DD YY   FROM   TO   MM DD YY

19. RESERVED FOR LOCAL USE

20. OUTSIDE LAB?   YES   NO $ CHARGES

21. DIAGNOSIS OR NATURE OF ILLNESS OR INJURY. (RELATE ITEMS 1,2,3 OR 4 TO ITEM 24E BY LINE)

1.   3.

2.   4.

22. MEDICAID RESUBMISSION CODE   ORIGINAL REF. NO.

23. PRIOR AUTHORIZATION NUMBER

24. A DATE(S) OF SERVICE From MM DD YY To MM DD YY	B Place of Service	C Type of Service	D PROCEDURES, SERVICES, OR SUPPLIES (Explain Unusual Circumstances) CPT/HCPCS MODIFIER	E DIAGNOSIS CODE	F $ CHARGES	G DAYS OR UNITS	H EPSDT Family Plan	I EMG	J COB	K RESERVED FOR LOCAL USE
1										
2										
3										
4										
5										
6										

25. FEDERAL TAX I.D. NUMBER   SSN EIN

26. PATIENT'S ACCOUNT NO.

27. ACCEPT ASSIGNMENT? (For govt. claims, see back)   YES   NO

28. TOTAL CHARGE $

29. AMOUNT PAID $

30. BALANCE DUE $

31. SIGNATURE OF PHYSICIAN OR SUPPLIER INCLUDING DEGREES OR CREDENTIALS (I certify that the statements on the reverse apply to this bill and are made a part thereof.)

SIGNED   DATE

32. NAME AND ADDRESS OF FACILITY WHERE SERVICES WERE RENDERED (If other than home or office)

33. PHYSICIAN'S, SUPPLIER'S BILLING NAME, ADDRESS, ZIP CODE & PHONE #

PIN#   GRP#

(APPROVED BY AMA COUNCIL ON MEDICAL SERVICE 8/88)   **PLEASE PRINT OR TYPE**

FORM HCFA-1500 (12-90),   FORM RRB-1500, FORM OWCP-1500

PATIENT AND INSURED INFORMATION

PHYSICIAN OR SUPPLIER INFORMATION

diagnostic codes and the CPT codes that are most commonly used in a specialty. The individual who completes the superbill simply checks off the procedure or procedures performed that day and places the charge for each service in the adjacent column. The superbill shows the amount due for services that day, any previous amount due, the payments made that day, and the total amount due.

For office-based practices, this method represented a way to a patient at the time of service and provided a form that could be used for insurance submittal. At the same time, it served as a receipt for patients who paid at the time of service. One of the biggest advantages of the superbill is that it can transfer the responsibility of collecting from third party insurance to the patient. Since superbills usually have three parts or more, one copy is given to the patient, a second copy serves as an encounter form for a patient's record, and the third is used by the business office or accounting clerk for post charges and payments. More often than not, posting goes to a ledger card with or without a pegboard, although some offices post directly to computer software. Although it certainly facilitated insurance processing, the superbill did little to help a practice in the overall control of the A/R, such as aging of the receivables.

Hospital-Based Physicians And Third Party Billing

Although the superbill was a great advantage for office-based practice, it did little to help the hospital-based physicians. In the early 1960s, several hospital-based disciplines, such as anesthesiology and radiology, moved to fee-for-service practices. This meant that rather than being an employee of the hospital and being paid by the hospital, these practitioners were responsible for billing patients and collecting for services. Some hospitals continued to do the billing for them, but others did not. Many hospital-based physicians did not want to get involved in the billing procedures. Thus, third party billing companies were formed to meet the needs of those physicians.

Choosing a third party biller is a business decision that requires the same care used in hiring an attorney or accountant. Third party billers run the gamut from individuals who provide a service out of the home to large corporations that specialize in this activity. A third party biller is a professional who has a great influence on the overall success of controlling A/R.

Since hospital-based physicians do not traditionally collect at the time of service, a need developed for an encounter slip to record the services they had rendered. This encounter slip or voucher transmits by paper, to the biller, information relative to the care that was rendered. In addition, encounter slips have to relay information to the biller about patient demographics as well as healthcare services rendered. In practices where the hospital does the billing, the hospital can rely on its own demographic database. As with any other aspect of billing, correct and accurate information is the basis of a successful outcome.

In-House Computer

With the declining cost of personal computers (PCs) and the increasing availability of software that can handle all aspects of managing A/R, more practices are turning to computer automation. The selection of an appropriate computer system is not an easy process. Anyone who has gone through the process of selecting, installing, and converting to a computer could write a book about it. It is rare to find people who feel they got everything they wanted, paid the amount they thought was appropriate, or didn't suffer during the conversion period. Some of the worst problems, however, have occurred in practices that for whatever reason have had conversions that were never quite right but have forged ahead anyway. Some of those practices are still feeling the effects of bad conversions that were done 5 years earlier.

A technological revolution has brought the PC into our everyday lives. Rapid changes have made terms such as "megabytes," "CD-ROM," "Prodigy," and "laptop" commonplace. Racks that once sported fishing and hunting magazines now carry a host of computer periodicals. I think it is important to understand the two aspects of buying a computer system: hardware and software. Hardware is the mechanical, physical part of a computer system; software refers to programs that process the data entered into the hardware.

In the 1970s and early 1980s there was only one way to have an automated system, and that was through the use of a midrange hardware system. However, as PCs grew in popularity, became more powerful, and required much smaller amounts of space, the practitioner ended up with a real option relative to hardware. However, it is important to remember that hardware is only the railroad track over which the data flow. What is important is the software that directs the data. As this book is being written, fee-for-service practices continue to be in a debit and credit environment. The growth in managed care has changed only the size of the discount that has to be added. However, if you look to the future relative to capitative care, the concept of the singular charge for a patient, a singular payment, and a singular write-off for managed care discount disappear. The type of software, not the hardware, will change immensely. Although it is hard to envision what's going to be necessary, it is safe to say that traditional software will be insufficient for these changes.

Making a Selection on the Basis of Price Alone

Selecting a computer system by price alone isn't the worst method, but price is not the only consideration and can lead to the purchase of a system that is not large enough for a practice, a system that is inefficient for a certain specialty, or a system without support. This brings to mind a practitioner I knew that was looking for a way to computerize his accounts receivable, but did not want to spend the money. He had a close friend who had developed an A/R billing system for an automobile tire store. The seller of the software persuaded the practitioner that it could be easily converted to his healthcare practice. As an example, he pointed out that when a CPT code was needed, the space available for the tire size could be utilized. Of course, the description of the tire would be the description of the medical service. However, inherent in the overall software was the singular choice, "with tube, or without tube." When the first statements were sent out, although there was adequate description of the services rendered and the amount owed, after each line entry was the phrase "with tube" or "without tube" appeared. You can image the dismay of the patients who received those statements. Those receiving statements for procedures such as "T & A" or "D & C" didn't question the nomenclature that followed, but you can image some of the questions about the other procedures.

An inexpensive computer system can also be detrimental when it comes to modification. When the concept of electronically submitted claims for Medicare was initiated, it rendered many systems obsolete because the software company couldn't or wouldn't produce the additional modifications necessary for true EMC submittal, or if they did, it charged exorbitant prices for the enhancement.

Understanding the Scope of What You are Doing

It is important to think through the total process of converting to a computer system before you begin. The needs for a very large group practice are different from those for a single practitioner. For example, a salesperson may sell a hardware system that should be sufficient to meet the needs of a very large practice. However, rarely does that salesperson mention that because of the number of monthly statements that will be produced, it is necessary to have a burster: a machine that separates the continuous forms and gets them ready for mailing. Something of this nature is not necessary for a solo practitioner. At the same time, a larger practice needs to purchase an inventory of a large number of forms to get them at discount prices, and this means finding space to store them. There are also other considerations in purchasing a computer, such as power surge protectors, laser printers, and modems. Inherent in all this is the financial side, such as the rate of depreciation of the hardware system and whether you are going to capitalize the software. Selecting the system is only a small part of the overall process.

In addition, thought has to be given to providing adequate space not just for the computer, but for computer supplies. Sufficient ventilation and cooling are needed, especially for large computer configurations. It is also important to consider backup and room for off-site storage of backup tapes. Most systems now mandate backup, but they can't make you take it off site. Remember that whatever is on that tape, disk, or diskette represents the entire financial side of your practice, and steps need to be taken to protect it.

Get Staff Members Involved in the Selection

In selecting a computer software system, it is extremely useful if the entire staff to participates in an open and frank discussion define its purpose now and in the future. For example, if you've been on a system that you've outgrown or one that couldn't be modified to keep up with regulatory and technological changes, individuals on your staff are going to provide a lot of input from their own perspective in regard to what you are looking for. If the previous system was used exclusively for billing and A/R management, staff members may suggest a system that also handles appointment scheduling: a medical office system (MOS). Perhaps over a period of time you started with one system for the billing and then bought another system for accounting, and it is now time to integrate both systems. Whether it's starting a new practice or combining several solo practitioners into a partnership, this means selecting a new system. Each participant has a different perception on what he or she needs.

Contact Other Users Before Buying

Probably one of the most important things you can do in considering a certain system is to contact other users. Ask who else is using the same software and whether you can contact them. You will probably be given a list of individuals to contact. At this point you will be tempted to call and ask them if they like the system you are considering purchasing. Invariably they will say yes, and the reason for that is simple. Software vendors often end up with a personable relationship with users. If the user is not satisfied, the salesperson is aware of it and is usually tries to ameliorate the situation. Since the purchasers are dependent on the salesperson's support, most likely they will not tell you if they are unhappy.

I suggest that you go beyond the general parameter of whether they are satisfied. Ask them what the program has done for the practice, what has it done for the analysis of A/R, and whether it has generated additional revenue for the practice. Finally, ask whether they got what they thought they would get and paid the price they thought they were going to pay. Did they end up with a lot of additional charges they weren't expecting? Did the conversion to the new system go as well as they expected? What did they encounter in that process?

Ask About User Groups

Be sure to ask the vendor whether there are user groups. A user group is a group of individuals who have the same or similar software and meet periodically to discuss how to get the most out of it. It is amazing what happens if you put a group of people in the same room, talking about the same software. By sharing ideas, they all have the potential to get the maximum benefits from the system. Ask the dealer if there are regular users group meetings, and if so, where are they held and when. Some user groups even have newsletters, so be sure to ask to get on the mailing list. Extra points should be given to any software vendor that has user groups within your locale. It brings forth a camaraderie that enables you to make the most out of the system and serves as a safety net.

The System Should have the Ability for Modification

If you believe that managed care is here to stay and that capitation will be part of it, the type of software needed will be significantly different. Although you can purchase a billing system off a shelf and save a substantial amount of money, what have you done to allow for the modification of that software as the changes take place in the healthcare delivery system? The onset of electronically submitted claims is an area where the ability for modification should be available. There are many more considerations to weigh, but remember the word "sophistication." The software must be sophisticated enough, and the hardware must be capable of being changed. Also think about what level of sophistication and support you want from your system relative to diagnostic and procedural coding. There are countless excellent programs that do coding checks relative to diagnostic codes and procedure codes. This type of software is particularly beneficial to practices that get large numbers of insurance rejections because the CPT code is not germane to the ICD-9 code. Any type of preedit in your software that ensures the outgoing claim not only is correct, but will meet the criteria for the prepayment audits run by the insurance company is very beneficial. If that is what you want, you have to remember to specify it.

Practice Analysis

Some computer software dump out so much practice analysis material that it may never be read or looked at. This is not to say that the practice analysis material available to a practitioner is not valuable. Some of it can be used in formulating managed care contracts and even managing the office for profitability. For example, a good practice management report is one that ranks CPT codes by frequency of use in descending order with average reimbursement by payer class. Many practice management consultants will tell you that's fantastic, but my hope is that you do not taking the time to look at this report every time you do a procedure to see which CPT code by payer class will get you the highest level of reimbursement. For most practices, just finding the time to work on the collection of the A/R is a challenge, without tracking this aspect of the A/R.

Another report may list CPT codes on the basis of the percentage of their collectibility. Although this is potentially a useful tool, let's hope that the patient receives the correct medical procedure even though it may be at the lower tier of collectibility. Be sure you not only understand the reports you are getting, but have a need for them. This is a way to save a couple of trees in your lifetime.

Training and Support

Two of the most important considerations in purchasing a software system are training of personnel and support from the software dealer after the training period is over. Most contracts for the purchase of software stipulate the number of hours or amount of training that your staff will be given. If they do not, ask the vendor how much training is included in the contract and what exactly will be covered in the training session. Will the training take place in your office, and if not, where will it take place? How many people can be trained?

Just as important is to find out whether the software company has technical support to answer questions if you run into a problem after the training is over. Ask if there is a charge for this support, and if so, how much. What hours during the week is support available? Many software firms maintain incoming toll free numbers which allow direct contact with a technician. Ask the vendor if the software offers "on-line" help screens, which provide instant answers. Technical support for software is very important and is a tremendous aid in helping you diagnose why the printer won't run or why specific reports can't be generated.

At a recent convention I attended I witnessed over 100 people buying into a bulletin board system despite knowing that there was no technical support and no toll free line; There was only a printed manual. Although a bulletin board system isn't very difficult to master, many of those people did not have the sophistication to handle even the slightest glitch. It is important to understand that you have to have some lifeline support, even if there is a charge for this service.

Retraining

You should look into the availability of retraining. Suppose the people who were initially trained on this system leave and new people are hired. If the system is complicated and the new staff members have no experience with it, a problem could be created if there is no retraining available. I know of a situation where staff members in a large group practice found in the training manual a way of putting a patient who had a problem or question about his or her statement on a hold status so the patient would not receive any more statements until the problem was resolved. When the office was very busy and came across a problem or dispute with a patient, it simply placed the patient's account on hold, hoping to get back to the problem in a short period. Each time they ran statements, they entered an exception code, and so a statement was not printed for that particular patient. It wasn't long before there were a number of patients who had unresolved problems with the practice but weren't asking questions because they weren't getting billed. For whatever reason, no one ever bothered to note on the computer instruction sheets that these accounts were being excluded from monthly billing. A new staff member started and followed the computer instruction sheet, printed the statements, and sent them out. Of course 3 days later the switchboard blew a fuse with a number of irate calls. I don't think there should be as much concern about the costs as long as retraining is available. Without this availability, your practice's A/R suffer.

Conversion Support

Whether you are going from one system to another or from a manual system to an automated one, conversion support is as important as the technical support you will need after the system is up and running. During the conversion it is possible that an immediate answer will have to be found for a specific problem. The basic question is whether someone will be with you or available at seven on Saturday night, when nothing seems to be going right. Along with availability is the question of cost: How much time will they give me for that conversion, and what will they charge me?

Hardware Maintenance and Disaster Support

After the system is functioning, proper training has taken place, and a successful conversion has been accomplished, there is still the question of maintaining the hardware and finding support if a catastrophe occurs. Ask the vendor who provides maintenance and at what cost. Sometimes a maintenance contract is offered. Ask what is included in the contract and what is not, such as lightening strikes or power problems. What is the extra charge for noncovered services? Does the maintenance contract cover services that are needed after hours or on weekends? If so, what are the rates? What kind of response time can your company guarantee for service calls?

Another type of support you should ask the vendor about is disaster support. As was mentioned earlier, most systems automatically demand some form of back up. Unfortunately, a total back up security system needs to be taken one step further. Ask the dealer how many users in your geographic area have the same system and are on the same configuration. In other words, even if you take the time to do all the right things and back up the system, your system may have a total breakdown. Where else can you run your software? Is there a neighboring physician who has excess computer time and the same configuration that you have who would allow you to get out your month-end statements? You may find the perfect system for your practice, but if you are the only user within a 50-mile radius and there is a disaster, there will be no way to run your software. Perhaps it is better to accept a less sophisticated system to ensure you have a disaster plan in effect.

Other Considerations In Purchasing a Computer System

Listed below are several other items worth investigation in researching and buying a computer system. Some may be of great importance to you and some may mean very little. They are presented as features to consider.

1. Can the system produce a bill for an entire family or just statements for each individual patient? Some software can handle either, but it is critical that the practice be able to describe the type of statement it wishes to send.

2. Who owns or has access to the source code? The source code is the original language that was used to create the software, and no alternation of your computer software can take place without it. Any acquisition of software without the source code can leave you totally dependent on the software vendor if you want to modify the program to deal with a new expectation or regulation change.

3. Does the software offer electronic claim processing? Almost all billing software packages today have some provision for electronic media claim submittal. Unfortunately, some of them are tied to only one clearinghouse, giving the user no options if a less expensive alternative becomes available. The availability of alternatives should be a key consideration.

4. Is the software user-friendly? A system that is user-friendly is one that is reasonably easy to use for someone without a lot of computer knowledge. When a computer package has all the bells and whistles, it may be too sophisticated for the average staff member to comprehend and use. Many of these packages have options, but if those alternatives are numerous that the left hand doesn't know what the right hand is doing, it won't be long before you have another challenge. This consideration is particularly important in practices where the turnover of personnel is high and retraining becomes necessary. Those tailored options won't gain you a thing if

extensive and comprehensive training is necessary before you can use them.

5. What added-value products are included? Does the system have word-processing capabilities? Does the software include Lotus or Excel, Windows or DOS? Is document imaging available with the package? Many modern packages include document imaging as part of the overall system. Document imaging is the easy recreation of a document on a computer for retrieval on demand. That technology coupled with the internal ability to transmit facsimiles can make most aspects of your practice much more efficient, but only if it is not going to cost a lot of additional dollars. If it's something the vendor is going to integrate into the cost of equipment, it definitely should be considered.

6. Can the system have multiple locations? Many systems were bought and installed for single-office use, and in a short time later the practice was operating multiple offices and couldn't interact with the other offices with the system it had.

7. Is there a security code feature that allows limited access to certain applications or files through the use of passwords? This can be a valuable asset for maintaining checks and balances. For example, each employee should be assigned a unique access code for the functions he or she needs to perform and should be able to have access only those specific functions. This also helps prevent collaboration among employees. One employee has an access code for posting payments to patient accounts, and another has a different access code to perform write-offs. These two employees cannot access each other's job function, and this makes for a fairly secure system of preventing embezzlement.

Request for Proposals (RFP)

One of the biggest problems in interviewing vendors for the selection of a computer A/R and billing system or a MOS is getting the same information so that a knowledgeable decision can be made by comparing apples to apples, rather than apples to oranges. Undoubtedly the best way to achieve that is by designing a written request for proposal (RFP). An RFP is a printed document that describes exactly what you need, what you want and when you want it. It is mailed to all the individuals who could fulfill that need, asking them to respond line for line to your RFP by a defined due date. When the RFPs are returned, you can make a chart or find another way to compare the answers you received. Appendix A shows a very elementary RFP for a computer system. An RFP should contain the following sections:

Section 1. A Profile of the Practice and A Description of What You Want.

It is important to tell the vendor exactly what type of practice you have. The RFP should include the type of discipline; the number of employees; the size of the practice, including the average number of patients seen monthly; the number of accounts billed monthly; and what kind of system the practice is currently using, whether manual or computer. This section also has to be very descriptive of your needs. You are telling the vendor what you want the system to do.

Section 2. A Profile of the Vendor's Company.

This section includes questions for the vendor to answer and blanks for the vendor to complete. This gives the salesperson a chance to brag about the company. If the vendor has brochures about his or her company, you should ask for them in the cover letter that you provide with the RFP. You want to ask how long the company has been in business, how many medical computer systems they installed last year, how many people are employed, and whether there is a list of references you can contact.

Section 3. Software Specifications.

Ask the questions about how the software being offered operates. List the specifications you want so they can tell you whether they have the capability. Ask if the system can provide an aging of A/R. Will the system produce Medicare and insurance claims? Does it have EMC capabilities? If you are looking for an MOS, insert questions about locating and updating patient records, automatic printout of patient files to be pulled, and the like. Also ask about technical support after the system is installed and training is over. Most important, what is the cost of this software?

Section 4. Hardware Specifications.

You need to know about the type of hardware the software will run on. Is the software best suited for specific hardware? Does the company sell the hardware? What is the cost? Is it also available for lease? What kind of warranties and support does the company provide? What additional equipment is included such as printers, modems, and terminals? What will the cost be for all items specified?

Section 5. Training and Maintenance.

The vendor should explain how much training it is going to provide and whether it will be on-site or off-site. How much is the charge for additional training? Are user groups available? Ask what type of maintenance contract the vendor can supply. How long does the original warranty last?

Each practice has different things in a computer system. Some practices want to know about the ability to expand or to connect to satellite offices. Others may need sophisticated word-processing programs because they do a lot of consultation work or medical writing. A large group practice may want to create separate files and reports for each physician with detailed month-end reporting. Asking vendor specific questions lets you compare the responses and weed out vendors that but have a product that does not supply what you need. The more candid the RFP, the better a final game plan.

Delegate Responsibility to the Conversion Team

During the process of selecting a computer system you need to consider your staffing. Whether for preparing and presenting RFPs, evaluating the proposals, or preparing for conversion, your office has to have some concept of who is going to be responsible for the overall undertaking. I cannot overemphasize the importance of an organizational chart showing who is responsible for each aspect of the conversion to a computer system. The members of the conversion team must have the power to make decisions. Many decision, big and small, need to be made during the conversion process. For example, suppose they discover an open account for a certain patient in the amount of $4. They need to have the right to write it off before it is converted into the new system. If all the decision making was your responsibility, you might end up with a successful conversion but you wouldn't be practicing medicine. Try to envision the overall process and delegate the responsibilities before you start.

Summary

To have good A/R management, an appropriate and proper billing system must be in place. There are many choices in the process of selecting one. The simplest and most economical is the use of a ledger card either with or without a pegboard or one-write system. A superbill which has preprinted detailed information such as CPT and ICD-9 codes not only provides detailed information in an easy to complete form but puts the burden of filing insurance claims onto the patient. However, the superbill does little without an A/R management system. Hospital-based physicians such as radiologists, anesthesiologists, and pathologists have a different challenge. Since they usually do not maintain medical offices as we know them and have gone to fee-for-service system, many have turned to professional billing companies to handle their billing and receivables.

With the continuously declining cost of computer hardware and the increasing availability of sophisticated software that can handle all aspects of billing and A/R management, more practices have turned to computerized billing. Selecting the proper type of computer software is an important endeavor and should be thoroughly examined. The decision should not be based solely on price. In fact, by getting the entire staff involved in the decision-making process, you can ensure that the practice will get exactly what it needs.

In requesting information from a dealer or vendor, there are important questions and features to consider. Get the names of other users and inquire about their overall satisfaction. Ask about training, technical support, and conversion assistance. Make sure the system is sophisticated enough to allow for modification, but not to the extent where one would need a degree in computer programming to run it. Ask about maintenance contracts and disaster support.

The best approach to buying a computer system is to prepare a request for proposal (RFP). Include information about the practice and be specific about what you are looking for. Get information about the vendor and his or her company. Include questions about the software specifications that you are looking for and the kind of hardware needed to run the software. Again, include questions about training, support, and hardware maintenance. After the choice has been made and the computer conversion process begins, delegate decision making to members of the conversion team. You'll end up with a computer system that will work efficiently for you and your practice.

CHAPTER 5

ORGANIZATIONAL NEEDS: JOB DESCRIPTIONS AND POLICY

In the management of A/R, one of the most important challenges a practice faces is taking care of its organizational needs, including managing its employees. One goal is to have personnel who perform with maximum productivity for the salaries they receive. To achieve this objective, it is important to hire competent people, give them precise job descriptions, properly train them, and then try to keep them on the payroll. At the same time you must organize the office using written and implicit policies and procedures.

Teamwork And The Problem Of Turnover

I have stressed the importance of making the staff in a practitioner's office feel like and function as a team, but building and creating a team are almost impossible without consistency among the players. Turnover of personnel is one of the biggest day-to-day challenges a medical practice faces in the overall management of A/R. Surveys conducted by the Practice Management Division of the American Medical Association found it is not uncommon for practices to have turnover of personnel every nine months. Other studies have shown that employee turnover rates: decrease as skill requirements of jobs increase; are higher among women than among men; are higher among married women than among single women; and differ widely between organizations. Although many practices can point with pride to long-term employees, practices that don't enjoy that status have a difficult challenge.

Maintain a Good Work Environment

There are many reasons for turnover of employees, including external events beyond the control of the practice. However, there are several things a practice can do to control this syndrome. Obviously, the work environment can be a critical factor. Is the office accessible by public transportation? What type of daycare is available, and what does it cost? Has the work environment been designed to be as stress-free as possible, including personal space? Providing a good work environment that is effective, efficient, and safe will enhance the overall productivity of your employees.

Instill a Sense of Value Through Recognition

Another element in achieving a sense of teamwork is whether an employee feels part of something special and feels appreciated and recognized. This appreciation can be achieved through formal and informal recognition. Formal recognition can be displayed by honoring the employee of the month with a plaque on the wall or a reserved parking space. Informally, recognition can consist of a pat on the back or a few nice words about the work that's been done. It is a natural human trait to want to be recognized.

Provide Continuing Education

A way to enhance team spirit is to provide continuing education. Continuing education comes in a variety of forms. Most Medicare intermediaries sponsor half-day or full-day seminars, usually by specialty. Not only does this demonstrate to employees that they are valued and that you want to train, it also allows them to get answers to specific problems your practice may be having relative to Medicare. Sometimes third party collection agencies sponsor informal meetings to discuss delinquencies and how to control them. It means time off from the job, but the benefits are twofold. It educates employees, enabling them to perform more knowledgeable services, and at the same time it tells them they are valuable to the practice.

Probably the most costly and time-consuming way to extend employee's continuing education is to provide continuing education at a local community college or vocational institute. The costs can be paid directly, or a reimbursement plan can be offered to employees once they have passed a course. Many community colleges offer courses in CPT and ICD-9 coding, computer classes, and accounting. Some even give A/R management courses. Yes, you may invest in tuition only to have an employee leave for a better job, but in the final analysis you are trying to tell your employees that you are willing to invest in them. It's a win-win situation for both the practice and the employee. The employee becomes more competent and knowledgeable in his or her job, which is a benefit to you, and at the same time retains a sense of self-esteem because he or she knows the practice wouldn't bother investing time or money in an employee that wasn't a valuable entity.

Attend Software User Meetings

Attendance at computer software user meetings is another way to build team spirit and receive added value in return. It often amazes me when a large office sends only one person to a software user meeting. Although I recognize the strain it places on the practice to send several people, the fact is that they are all users and could gain from such a program. How often have you rescheduled patients to provide yourself a free morning or afternoon? Isn't it possible to do the same for staff members?

Add Some Fun to the Workload

Another form of recognition, appreciation, and team awareness consists of having fun at group functions such as potluck lunches, field trips to a ball game, or another special event. It is not something that should be overdone, but if everyone gets a chance to let his or her hair down, relax a bit, and get to know the others better, it can be very beneficial in building a team. This type of undertaking can be particularly important to practices that have multiple offices where the staff members never get to interact with each other face to face.

Several years ago my company had grown quite large, and we had personnel in two buildings about two blocks apart. The majority of the employees knew each other by phone, but some had never met personally. We recognized the problem in mid-September and decided to have an Octoberfest in the parking lot of one of the buildings. I became the chef and cooked for the entire staff. It was a bit reminiscent of an eighth grade dance: the employees from one building stayed on one side of the parking lot and the employees from the other building stayed on the other side. The next year, we opted to hold another Octoberfest, and this time everyone seemed to loosen up and have a good time. Team spirit was back again. In fact, it became a tradition at our company.

However, after awhile a few employees questioned why we were holding a festival honoring one nationality, so instead of Octoberfest we now pick a local event one without a lot of cost, such as a ball game, and anyone who wants to attend can bring family members, spouses, or guests. Attendance varies, but we always end up having a great time. There are other benefits to these functions, such as the chance to meet an employee's family and learn more about them personally, which will often give you an opportunity to learn about the motivators in your employees' lives. Again, one of the most advantageous outcomes of enjoyable group activities is the feeling of team spirit they bring.

Job Descriptions

There are some other basic considerations that must be present in a team relationship. First and foremost is letting team players know exactly what is expected by using an explicit job description. Written job descriptions should always end with words such as, "and whatever other responsibilities are assigned from time to time." In today's world, we must include disclaimers in almost everything we do because of continuing federal mandates and case law. It's good business sense to have everything open and thoroughly understood from the very beginning.

A well-written job description identifies for both the employer and the employee the level of responsibility and type of work expected. Figure

5-1 shows a job description for a receptionist. For example, you hire an individual for a receptionist's position and then ask that person to make phone calls to patients who are delinquent. If that individual has no training, there probably will be a high level of dissatisfaction. Unfortunately, some people accept an employment position on the basis of the original job description they received and do not wish to expand or learn new functions. Of course there are people who thrive on

Figure 5-1: Sample job description

Job Description for a Receptionist

Job Title: Receptionist

Supervisor: Office Manager

SUMMARY

The primary purpose of the receptionist's job is to serve as the intermediary between this office and the outside world as people arrive in person or call on the telephone.

DUTIES

    1. Have a sign-in chart prepared daily.

    2. Ask patients to sign in as they arrive

    3. Ask each new patient to complete a patient information sheet.

    4. As returning patients to complete a patient update sheet.

    5. As patients exit, prepare charge slips and ask for payment.

    6. Answer all incoming telephone calls.

    7. When necessary, take detailed messages.

    8. Straighten magazines in waiting room.

    9. Do other duties at the request of the office manager.

QUALIFICATIONS

    1. High school graduate

    2. Self-starter, able to work without constant supervision

    3. Good telephone manner

    4. Neat appearance

WORK SCHEDULE

Monday, Tuesday, and Thursday: 9:00a.m.-5:00p.m.

Wednesday: 12:00p.m.-7:00p.m.

Friday: 9:00a.m.-7:00p.m.

First and third Saturdays: 9:00a.m.-12:00p.m.

learning everything they can and function well under constant changes in responsibility, but they are in the minority. If your office has a tendency to shift duties and expand responsibilities, it is important to add a brief statement to a job description saying that the functions of the job may change from time to time with the needs of the practice.

The job description should also specify the work hours. If that is impossible because of fluctuations in the practice, that should be stated. An individual who takes a job and perceives that the weekday will end at 3:30 p.m. each day usually plans her family life around it. She will probably turn in her resignation when she learns that departure at that time every day is impossible. Also, either in the job description or in an office policy handbook, there should be a statement regarding the employee's performance review, how often it is done, and what factors will be used in that review. Once this is specified, it should be adhered to. As with most interactions between employer and employee, a review should be in writing with room for the employee to acknowledge by countersigning it. A job evaluation lets the employee know how he or she is doing and what can be done to improve performance, and also allows the manager or practitioner to know more about the employee and possibly how to improve or streamline some of the tasks involved.

Once the job description is complete and agreed on by all parties, an activity sheet can be prepared for the employee. An activity sheet specifies each duty and when it should be done, such as daily, weekly, monthly, or annually. Because it spells out each duty, this becomes a double-check system to ensure that every chore is covered and indicate who is responsible for it. It also helps if someone is out sick or on vacation. An activity sheet is a helpful tool for a practice. Figure 5-2 shows an activity sheet for a medical assistant in a one-person office. Job descriptions and activity sheets are not an easy undertaking in a busy healthcare practice, but without them, there is no way to assign individual responsibilities and duties, especially as they relate to your accounts receivable.

Background Checks And Fiduciary Responsibility

Interviews I have had with practice management consultants show a consistency in their belief that 60 percent of medical practices suffer from embezzlement at some point. The majority of those crimes go unreported for a host of reasons. The first the most common reason is that the practitioner fails to take the time and/or use outside expertise to document the problem for further action. The second reason, which ties in with the first, is that people do not want to acknowledge that they've been taken. In many cases, they cannot justify the amount of money stolen and the time and court cost it will take to recover it. Therefore, it is possible to interview a perspective employee with a letter of recommendation from a previous job in the healthcare field and still not have complete confidence in the applicant's character. For that reason, great effort and care should be used in hiring, and one should require that the perspective employee allow a credit bureau check or that the applicant's references be checked beforehand.

Consequently, it is important for a practice to ensure that checks and balances are in place to reduce the incidence of that type of situation.

Figure 5-2: Sample activity sheet

Activity Sheet for Medical Assistant

Daily Duties   Sequence

Open and handle incoming mail   _____
Tidy the office   _____
Check supplies   _____
Sterilize equipment as necessary   _____
Check daily roster of patients   _____
Have new patients complete information sheet   _____
Escort patients to examining room   _____
Check blood pressure and weight as necessary   _____
Assist physician as required   _____
Prepare examining rooms after each appointment   _____
Prepare bill for services and collect from patient   _____
Arrange for additional tests for patients   _____
Arrange for hospital admissions   _____
Post charges and payments   _____
File insurance as required   _____
Make entries into patients' records and refile folders _____
Pull charts for the next day   _____
Call patients for the next day's appointments   _____
Prepare bank deposits   _____

Weekly Duties

Pay incoming bills
Order supplies as necessary
Call past-due accounts

Monthly Duties

Prepare and send statements
Prepare month-end reports
Reconcile office checkbook

Yearly Duties

Gather information on accounts for tax purposes
Prepare and send holiday cards
Sort through files and store old records

The method of checks and balances varies with the type of practice, but in a traditional office practice where a day sheet is used, it needs to be balanced at the conclusion of each workday, not 2 or 3 days later. One of the items that needs to be balanced daily is the number of charge tickets or encounter forms that were issued during the day and whether they matched the day sheet. Periodic checks should also include whether all charges were posted to the billing system and whether all receipts, including cash, credit card slips, and checks, were properly posted and accounted for. Many computer programs have checks and balances built in, but a practice does have exposure, and appropriate steps need to be taken to test that exposure periodically.

In some instances, consideration should be given to the value of a fiduciary bond to cover the misuse of income. A fiduciary bond is an insurance policy that pays for the recovery of funds if proceeds are lost because of employee dishonesty, rather than relying on the ability of the employee to repay the loss. Normally this type of bond is inexpensive and can also be used as a hiring tool. If you establish a policy by which each applicant is required to be bonded, you can ask potential employees during the interview session or on the employment application whether they are bondable. It is surprising how many people asked that question don't return for the second interview.

Policy Handbook

An employee or policy handbook may not stop turnover, but it will reduce repetitive debates between employer and employee. All aspects of employment should be included in a clear and precise manner. The use of such a book also helps reduce misunderstandings and claims for unemployment. However, be aware that employee policy manuals and handbooks can be the basis a lawsuit. In many states, the courts have upheld the notion that an employee handbook may constitute a legal contract that is binding on the employer. In some cases, employees have sued their employers for breach of contract or wrongful discharge when the employer failed to comply with the terms of the handbook. As a precaution, be sure to add disclaimers to the handbook that clearly deny any contractual relationship and do not suggest anywhere in the book that there is an express or implied contract.

Attendance and Tardiness

An employee handbook should include a statement of policy regarding attendance and tardiness. The absence of such a statement suggests that absenteeism and tardiness are never going to be problems and therefore don't have to be addressed, which is illogical, or that they don't matter. Whether an employee is penalized is a matter of choice, but every minute that is lost is a reduction of the time spent on A/R management. A few quick calls to colleagues may give you an idea of the prevailing policies in the immediate area. A practice's position on vacation days, sick days, and holidays is also critical and should be spelled out.

Employee Benefits

Employee benefits are not supposed to be rewards for performance; rather they are a package of added-value features that supplement an employee's compensation. Although they help create a secure and productive environment for employees, they also must be cost-effective and easily administered. Some employee benefits are legally required, such as Social Security, worker's compensation, and unemployment insurance. Optional benefits include group health insurance, disability and life insurance, pension plans, thrift incentive plans, and individual retirement accounts (IRAs).

Employee benefits should be clearly specified in writing, usually in the policy handbook. If health insurance benefits are available to full-time employees, provide information about what those benefits include, what percentage the employee pays and what percentage the employer pays, and how much it will cost for dependent coverage. In larger

Figure 5-3: Sample organizational chart

Organization Chart for the Practice of Richard M. Patton M.D.

Dr. Patton

Medical Assistant
Prep exam room
Escort patients
Take vitals
Assist Doctor
Screen phone calls

Office Manager
Oversee all operations
Oversee all personnel
Order supplies
Phone delinquent accounts
Back up medical assistant

Receptionist
Prepare sign-in sheets
Pull charts
Register patients
Answer phones
Prepare charge slips
Issue receipts

Book Keeper
Post charges
Post payments
Balance daily
Make deposits
Prepare reports
Back up ins. clerk

Typist/Ins. Clerk
Transcribe notes to charts
Complete insurance forms
Follow-up with insurance
Back up receptionist

practices, there may be more than one option available, such as choosing between a Health Maintenance Organization (HMO) or a standard health insurance policy. In any case, it is important that the employee understands exactly when the insurance goes into effect and how much it will cost, and receive a pamphlet or booklet describing the benefits of the program. Also, make sure you update your policy handbook if there are changes because you don't want to have a statement in the handbook which is not consistent with the health insurance plan.

Another benefit to consider is providing uniform allowances. If this option is chosen, give specific information about how the program works and its dollar value. Other items that may be considered include offering floating personal days off, paid memberships in professional trade associations, the ability to join a credit union, and scholarships for dependent children. In some situations (although this should not be included in your office policy manual), you might supply free lunch. This can help overcome the problem of keeping staff members happy when things are hectic and you can't guarantee a specific lunch break. Once again you are building team spirit by recognizing the inconveniences inherent in the job.

Dress Code

If a practice does not require uniforms, some sort or written or implicitly understood dress code should be established. It would be nice if every employee arrived at work wearing clothing appropriate for the job, but that doesn't always happen. The words "appropriate dress" can cover a lot of ground, so if and when that fateful day comes, you can simply counsel the employee about why the attire was inappropriate.

Organizational Chart

Besides a written policy manual for employees, another item should be a part of the overall operation of a practice: an organizational chart. This can be a simple piece of paper or a detailed graph, but it should show who is accountable for each aspect of the work that needs to be done and the chain of command for that process. It also should indicate who is available as the backup for each duty in the office. This document deserves a lot of thought because it ultimately will spell out what every employee can and cannot do. It will serve as a road map that depicts exactly what you are and are not willing to delegate.

The organizational chart actually represents a coordination of each job description and how these descriptions relate to each other and to the overall operation of a practice, especially in regard to the management of an A/R. Some of the elements that should be included are assignments of responsibility for confirming appointments 24 hours in advance, who is responsible for asking for payment at the time of service, and who is ultimately responsible for ensuring that timelines (such as prompt billing and prompt insurance filing) take place. Figure 5-3 shows an organizational chart for a small, one-physician office.

Patient Brochures

Just as employees need to know exactly what they can expect in regard to compensation, benefits, duties, and how they fit into a practice, patients need to know how they can get answers and be informed about what is expected of them. This can best be accomplished through patient brochures.

Patient brochures are marketing tools, but they can also do much to reduce needless interruptions of your staff. A patient brochure should introduce the practitioner and key staff members to new patients so that the patients know who to contact relative to any questions they have. It can include a policy on collecting payment at the time of service, how Medicare and insurance claims are handled, and what a patient should do if he or she cannot make a scheduled appointment. It normally specifies office hours, who to call in an emergency, and depending on the discipline of the practice, various medical warning signs of which the patient should be aware, along with instructions on what to do and who to call in those cases.

Credit Policy

Every time you extend medical care, you are extending unsecured credit. Whether or not it is included in the patient brochure, every medical office should have a written credit policy so that all patients (and employees), know exactly what is expected regarding financial indebtedness. A clearly defined and understood policy will have a positive effect on a practice's A/R. A credit policy can be as brief or as extensive as desired, but it should inform patients about customary credit procedures and tell them that payment is expected at time of service. It should include a statement that tells patients about their financial responsibility and about the efforts that will be undertaken if an obligation is not met in a timely manner, such as referral to a third party collection agency. In addition, if there is a fee for broken appointments, it should be included in the credit policy. However, first and foremost a credit policy should state that your primary purpose is to provide medical care on the basis of need and that no other consideration will govern the quality of the medical care you provide. An sample credit policy is shown in Figure 5-4.

Figure 5-4: Sample written credit policy

Credit Policy of Family Medical Practice

☑ Your health is first and foremost. Medical care will always be rendered solely on the basis of need, and no other factor will affect the quality of that care.

☑ Payment is expected at the time of service.

☑ For patients who are unable to pay at the time of service, we are always willing to consider special arrangements for payment.

☑ Patients who are financially unable to pay will be given special consideration. Please make an appointment to speak with the accounts receivable manager, Deborah.

☑ In fairness to our patients who do pay, after reasonable efforts on our part to obtain payment, we will solicit the services of a collection agency if necessary.

Internal Policy on Partial Payments

A policy on partial payments should be part of your internal credit policy but does not have to be included in the patient brochure. Of course, changes and deviations can always be made, but without a policy there is no uniformity or consistency. Patients who request and end up on a payment plan can have a dramatic effect on the management of receivables because there is more work involved in keeping track of and administering a payment plan. Worse yet are patients who never ask for a payment plan but simply inflict one on a practice. A patient who owes $200 and without any discussion or permission starts sending $10 a month has a pretty good deal. However, if a practice ends up with a large number of these payment plans, managing A/R and trying to keep within the target numbers will become increasingly difficult.

This brings to mind an obstetric practice in which, after the delivery of the first child, the mother began sending small monthly payments. In subsequent years the same woman delivered eight more children, but never varied her payment plan. The end result was that the practice had a receivable that was over $18,000 and was being paid off at $25 a month. If one staff member is accepting $5 a month and another is demanding 20 percent of the balance every month, there is no consistency. A written partial payment policy makes it easier for front desk employees to deal with a patient who, because of financial circumstances, must make payments on some sort of payment plan. If the patient is there in person, the policy can be handed to him, or it can be sent if communication is done by phone or mail. In any case, establish a payment plan that will be reasonable for the patient but satisfy the debt in a timely manner. There is no single-best plan and dollar amounts vary with the type of discipline, but keep in mind the fact that even a plan that mandates 20 percent of the balance will keep an account open for an additional 150 days. If you are trying to get your days outstanding in the 60-day range, a few payment plans at 20 percent can make that job difficult. Figure 5-5 shows a written partial payment policy.

Internal Policy on Sending Accounts for Collection

An internal credit policy should go one step further by telling staff members under what circumstances and in what time frame an account should go to collection and whether this must be authorized by the practitioner. Please remember that if you give your staff the responsibility of reducing the days outstanding on you're a/R but insist that every account be authorized by you before going to collection and then let the papers sit on your desk for 30 days, you are defeating the purpose and telling your staff that the plan won't work. You have to be a team player too and work with them to achieve the goals that you have set.

In terms of an actual policy for sending accounts to collection agencies, timelines vary according to the type of specialty and the strength of

Figure 5-5: Sample partial payment policy statement

Policy Statement Regarding Partial Payment to the Practice of _____.

It is recognized that from time to time patients will make requests for partial payment plans. Please adhere to the following policy.

1. Ascertain why the payment plan is necessary. Recognize that unemployment may necessitate a more liberal plan.

2. Balance over $750: 15 percent of balance every 30 days. If in default for 1 month, account goes to collection.

3. Balance under $750: 20 percent of balance every 30 days. If in default for 1 month, account goes to collection.

---

your desire for good public relations. As a guideline, though, it should be an emulation of the A/R ratio that is the eventual goal. If you are trying to maintain a ratio of 3:1 or below, the policy should specify review of an account for collection at 90 days. Again, there may be variations on the basis of financial class, but if the majority of accounts linger for 120 to 150 days before being considered for collection, it is unlikely that a 3:1 ratio will be achieved. An internal policy statement helps the entire staff understand what you are trying to achieve and gives the staff backup when you are not there.

Policy Toward Accepting New Patients

Another important consideration for effective teamwork and ultimate management of receivables is your policy on accepting new patients. Your staff members have to have an understanding of what you expect them to do when they get a call for an appointment from a new patient who is clearly going to be in the financial category of self-pay. Although you expect employees to book all new appointments without consideration for financial class, you need to ask your staff to tell the patient what the expected charge will be, explain that payment is expected at the time of service, and state your policy on insurance filing and Medicare assignments. This will help set things straight in the beginning and clear a path for smooth collection efforts in the future.

Summary

To manage receivables effectively, a practice must know how to manage its personnel. Ideally, a practice strives to hire competent individuals and keep them as long as they perform effectively. It is to the advantage of a practice to have the entire staff function as a team. By working together as a team, employees get a better feeling of their individual worth and are more willing to work hard. Turnover is detrimental to the management of receivables. There are many ways to prevent of turnover, such as formal and informal types of recognition. These includes special privileges, plaques on the wall, and verbal acknowledgment. Continuing education, whether at a local community college, at a seminar, or in an informal session with a vendor, helps instill a feeling of team spirit and self-worth in employees.

For an office to run with the least level of friction, a practice should use written job descriptions that spell out the duties of each position. A clearly defined organization chart should be designed so all employees know their responsibilities and the order of command, and appropriate backup is available. To protect the practice, time should be spent examining a potential employee's background, and making sure checks and balances are in place regarding fiduciary responsibilities.

In addition, to reduce misunderstandings about policies within the practice, a handbook should be provided that states policies on attendance and tardiness, employee benefits, and the dress code. For clear communication with new and returning patients, it is advisable to provide a friendly but clearly stated patient brochure that introduces the practice and advises patients about office hours, what to do in an emergency, and the practice's policy on extending credit. A written credit policy for both staff members and patients will help ensure that the office will function on a level that will maximize the well-being of both the practice and the A/R.

CHAPTER 6

PERCEPTION IS REALITY

Responsible people pay their bills because it is their obligation and the honorable thing to do. However, a concept known as diminishing appreciation can affect a physician's A/R. The longer the lapse between the time a service is rendered and the time a bill is presented to the recipient of that service, the less desire there is to pay for the service. Thus, appreciation diminishes as time increases. Therefore, a positive perception from the onset can enhance that gratitude. People sometimes look for reasons not to pay a bill.

On the day a patient is treated, his or her desire to pay is in most cases 100 percent, provided that the patient know's who you are, what you did, and why it was important. Whether you relieve pain, remove anxiety, or lay out a course of treatment that will correct a problem, as long as what you did is known to the patient, he will have a strong desire to pay you. However, every day thereafter, that desire diminishes and in the process, patients take on defensive or negative mind-sets in regard to why they shouldn't pay or why it is not their responsibility. The change in perspective from positive to negative is usually illogical and unfounded, but since perception is reality, it is critical to keep that perception positive. Perceptions are like first impressions. More often than not, a practice that has not presented a positive image of its staff, its care, and its overall image will have a large problem with it's a/R management.

Some practices consistently do better than others. Why is this so? The answer is not always found in the overall management of receivables, but rather in something more subtle. This chapter will deal with some of the extra things that can make a practice more successful. Part of it is going the extra mile, and part of it is simply presenting a better impression to patients. Many patients perceive something that may not be quite factual, but nevertheless it is real to them.

Going A Step Beyond

By going an extra step, one physician can have a more successful practice than another even though both are in the same specialty and locale. An example of this occurred with four anesthesiologists working independently at the same hospital, with each physician scheduled for one week of work per month. As a result, they all had basically the same patient financial mix. Each used the same third party medical billing system, which handled their A/R management identically. One physician approached the billing company and asked what he could do to increase his collections. The recommendation was that when doing post-operative visits, he leave his business card, as all the anesthesiologists did on the preoperative visit. Their rationale was that the stronger the name identification, the better the patient will recognize the name when the bill is received. Invariably, this physician's practice began collecting a minimum of 3 percent more than did his peers.

Enthralled with the success of this program, he returned to the billing office and asked for other suggestions. They recommended that he do two postoperative visits, recognizing that during the first visit the patient would still be feeling the effects of the anesthesia. Although the business card was having an effect, it was probably due to the presence of family members. This physician then worked out a schedule that allowed him to call on the majority of his patients a second time, normally on the day of discharge. Although this created additional work, he witnessed a consistent collection recovery that was at least 7 percent higher than that of his peers. In most cases an anesthesiologist doesn't have much face-to-face contact with patients, so anything that reinforces the fact that the anesthesiologist performed a valuable service and has a very deep concern for the patient's well-being helps when it comes time for the patient to pay the bill.

What Message Are You Giving Your Patients?

I have been working with an obstetric-gynecologic practice that for the past six years has had an ongoing problem managing its receivables. Although countless problems have been diagnosed and each one corrected, the practice still has a long way to go. Before the entire overhaul is finished, we will probably find that the interior designer played a small role in the problem. There is no question that when the waiting room was designed, it was extremely attractive and appealing to patients. Unfortunately, every piece of furniture in the waiting room was done in fabric, even though the practice knew that its patients would often come with small children.

Because the practice was having economic problems, it failed to focus on maintaining a new look in the waiting room. As time went by, almost every chair and couch became well worn and soiled. Although I may be stretching the point here, I suspect that if we really got down to the bottom line and interviewed the patients who were not paying their bills, some of the objections and reasons would relate to their feeling that the practice doesn't care about them. Therefore, why should they care about the practice?

Conversely, I know a dentist who invariably is always running a few minutes behind. As much as everyone hates going to the dentist, I've got to hand it to him. He recognizes the importance of not only having current magazines in the lobby, but having interesting magazines, that usually aren't available in waiting rooms. The magazines he has are different and interesting to the point where patients almost hope he will run late so that they'll have a chance to scan the current *Smithsonian*.

By contrast, there is an endodontist who is well known and has a very busy practice. However, something is lacking in the diplomacy department. Within seconds after the first treatment, patients are forced to listen and respond to an explanation of estimated costs and payment expectations. Written information is also supplied, but often it is much more tactful to talk about payment at a time when the patient isn't suffering from the trauma of the first appointment.

Patient-Friendly Guidelines For The Office

Below are some guidelines for presenting a good first impression of a practice that can ultimately help in the overall management of receivables by reflecting the practice's concern for its patients.

Furniture

Although the type of practice often dictates the nature of the waiting room and examining rooms, emphasis should be placed on material that is stain-resistant and comfortable. For example, couches look inviting until three people are forced to sit shoulder to shoulder. This can be an awkward and uneasy situation for most patients. With the idea of practical yet comfortable furniture comes the desire for personal space. Twenty-five identical chairs placed so that all the patients are staring at each other do not afford that luxury.

Color, Sound and Soothing Effects

In most cases patients come to a physician because they have a problem. Often they don't feel well. Therefore, the use of color as a calming and comforting mechanism is important, along with the type of background music and anything else you do to take patients' minds off their problems.

Let me describe a practice setting to make my point clear. A fertility clinic is located in a modern and spacious professional building. Its offices are on the first floor in a secluded area. Obviously, patients coming to such a practice are in desperate need of help. However, as you enter, the first sound you hear is hard rock music because that's what the office manager likes. The furniture is a collection from three practices that have merged, and the music seems to increase the clashing of the colors. In the center of the waiting room is a massive aquarium. Unfortunately, it's stocked not with rare exotic fish of many colors, but several carnivorous species known to eat smaller fish. Some shortcuts were taken in construction also. Hollow-core doors are substantially cheaper than solid doors, but cost shouldn't be a determining factor, particularly when the doors are on examining rooms. Anyone who designs a pediatrician's office knows that the outlets should be 30 inches off the floor. Shouldn't the same go for the design of an obstetrician's office, where there will be small children at times? In this case, the outlets were just above the baseboards. This may sound overly subtle, but we are also dealing with an obstetric patient who says she doesn't want to pay her bill because she feels her child was endangered.

Layout

There is a very successful orthopedic practice in a midwestern community that has gained an incredible reputation for joint replacements. However, the entrance to the waiting room is through two double sets of doors that are not electrically assisted, making access for patients in wheelchairs or with walkers almost impossible. The waiting room has 47 individual chairs, but the aisle space is the exact width of a standard wheelchair. In essence, if a patient in a wheelchair gets into the back of the waiting room and then has to be moved to an examining room, all the other patients sitting in that aisle must get up and move. With that kind of commotion, it's no wonder that patients do not want an afternoon appointment because by that time, the office is running at least an hour behind. Patients who feel put down in this manner are often the ones who don't pay their bills in a timely fashion.

Provide A Quiet Place To Talk To Patients About The Bill

One of the most overlooked design factors involves ensuring that staff members have a designated space to talk quiet and privately to patients about their bills and ask for payment at the time of service. Money is a very personal subject, and there is a far better chance that you will get the real story if it is talked about in semi-privacy. This is helpful for staff members also. Picture a staff member asking a patient for payment through a glass cubbyhole with the patient standing among all the patients who are still waiting. If that patient evades the request, it is quite likely that other patients who overhear the conversation will do the same. Conversely, if quiet space has been provided, only two parties would have known who won or lost the war. Quiet space doesn't mean bringing the patient back into the business office with all the distractions of other staff members going about their duties. Quiet space consists of an area removed from all patients and staff, where your staff member and the patient can have a focused discussion without disruptions.

Summary

Patients usually appreciate what you have done for them and have a real desire to pay their bills. However, that appreciation diminishes as time passes. As time goes by, patients look for reasons not to pay their bills. If they perceive that a practice and a practice setting don't look to their needs, it is real to them and consequently, their desire to pay may reflect those feelings. The difference between a successfully run practice and one that is not so successful can depend on going a step further.

When a patient comes to you for treatment, his or her first impression of your practice will most likely be a lasting one. You need to create a setting that says you care with comfortable furniture arranged to provide adequate personal space. Colors and music should be delicately handled to create a soothing and relaxing atmosphere. In busy practices where there are sometimes long waits, it is important to create a waiting room that is pleasing to patients and gives them things to do or read that are different, interesting, or unusual. All these factors can make the difference between a totally satisfied patient and one who is not enthralled, and can affect a patient's attitude toward paying the bill.

In addition, a practice should provide quiet space for communication between staff members and patients about their bills. A little diplomacy and tactfulness during the explanation of charges and expected payment goes a long way. Reinforce your overall policy through the use of laminated signs that state that payment is expected at the time of service. A sign of this nature, along with a patient brochure reinforcing the message, should make your staff members feel better about asking for payment at the time of service.

You need to make sure that incoming calls are handled in an efficient manner by ensuring that the caller is connected without delay to the staff member who can best help him. If a patient with a delinquent bill calls and is put on hold, there is an excellent chance that he or she will hang up; after all, the patient tried to tell the doctor that he or she was paying but couldn't get through. Don't give a patient an opportunity to conjure an illogical perception of why he or she shouldn't pay. As insignificant as some of these things may seem, they portray an attitude to patients who, in turn, take that perception and turn it into reality.

CHAPTER 7

USE OF THE TELEPHONE AND OTHER TOOLS IN A/R MANAGEMENT

In the management of receivables, there are three methods for communicating with patients in regard to their financial obligations to a practice: face-to-face conversation, the written word, and the telephone. The most effective is verbal communication done in person. However, this opportunity usually is present only when a patient is physically in your presence. In a perfect world, this is the time and place for securing all the demographic information, explaining payment policies, and collecting for services. Unfortunately, few practices function in a perfect world. In all probability further steps will have to be taken to secure payment for your services.

The second method for communicating with patients about indebtedness is the written word. You send statements to patients who have open balances on you're a/R and add a message that lets them know you expect payment. This form of communication is discussed in Chapter 3. Although the written word conveys your message, it does not create a sense of urgency.

The third vehicle is communication with patients by telephone. The telephone is a valuable and inexpensive tool, yet in many practices the person using that device has never had any instruction on how to use it efficiently and successfully. Many ingredients are helpful in making two-way communication on the telephone effective. They include proper planning, maintaining a positive mental attitude, keeping control of the situation, listening to what the patient is saying, and closing the deal.

Plan Appropriately

Before making a call to a patient who has not paid a bill, it is important to do a quick review of that person. Quickly go over his chart and note such things as his age, marital status, where he works and what the bill was for. By becoming familiar with the patient's situation, you can quickly and accurately handle questions or objections the patient might have. Look at the amount due and establish a mental goal for what you want to accomplish with the phone call. If the balance is very high, consult your partial payment policy so that you can negotiate a payment plan if payment in full is not possible. The ultimate goal in making a collection call is payment in full (PIF), but that's not always possible. Be prepared with your questions. You may need information about the patient's insurance and whether there is a new address or phone number. To be effective, you must be confident, knowledgeable, and organized.

Maintain A Positive Attitude

A positive mental attitude (PMA) is important in achieving success in all walks of life. When you have a PMA, an image is reflected in your voice and manner that conveys to the recipient of the call that you are confident about what you are doing. When you telephone a delinquent debtor, you are assuming that: (1) the patient owes the practice money; and (2) the patient will pay the bill. Keep a PMA and the result will often be payment of the account.

Keep Control Of The Situation

A patient who owes a practice money is not going to enjoy receiving a call about the situation. The caller must maintain control of the call by adopting a polite but firm manner. A collection call should be direct and simple, and should be made with confidence. If the patient becomes argumentative or angry, the caller should remember not to take it personally. The patient is not angry at the collection clerk who is calling, but at the situation the clerk represents. If a patient uses profanities or obscenities, the clerk should say something like, "Mr. Jones, I do not have to listen to language like this. I will call you another day." If the clerk lets the patient take control of the call, the chance of having a successful conclusion is minimal.

Listen

Listening is extremely important in a collection telephone call. Really listen to the speaker and don't interrupt or change the topic unless the speaker gets off the subject—payment in full. Ask questions when necessary and be responsive to the patient's questions or objections. If you ask a patient to send payment in full now and then pause to listen to his remarks, you will most likely learn what the real problem is and will be better able to find a solution. If you say little and listen a lot, the patient may find the solution to his own problem, leading to payment in full or a payment plan and a constructive conclusion.

Close The Deal

Like a salesperson who tries to get a customer to buy something, a person making a collection call is trying to "sell" the patient on paying the bill. If you have accurate information and approach the situation in a positive manner, a solution usually can be negotiated. An agreement must be made for the amount of payment and the date when it will be made. Be specific. Repeat the amount and date back to the patient so that everything is clear: "Then you will mail us a check for $150 on April 12 and the balance of $100 on May 12." You should even ask the patient to repeat the agreement so that everyone understands it. Be sure to note the results in the chart for future follow-up, which usually won't be necessary.

Seven Steps To A Successful Collection Phone Call

A successful collector is very much aware of and trained in the following seven steps for a successful collection phone call. I've modified these steps somewhat for a medical office, but the basic principals are the same. They incorporate the factors we have already discussed: proper planning, maintaining a positive mental attitude, keeping control, listening, and closing the deal. These steps have proven to be effective because they provide a psychological edge over the party you are contacting about a debt. Figure 7-1 provides helpful reminders of some things you should and should not do when making a collection call.

Step 1. Identify the person you are calling

> *"Hello. Is this George Smith?"*
>
> *"Yes, it is."*

Before you tell the patient who is calling, identify the party you are trying to reach. You want to be sure you are talking to the right person. If you are calling a George Smith III, you should ask who you are speaking to. Also, once a patient knows who's calling, he or she may become a different party. Finally, even though a physician's office is not covered under the Federal Debt Collection Practices Act (FDCPA), disclosure to a third party regarding another person's delinquency isn't a good practice. It's a private matter between the physician's office and the person who owes the debt.

Step 2. Identify yourself

> *"Mr. Smith, my name is Jennifer Jones, and I am the accounts receivable manager for Dr. Martin Johnson. Dr. Johnson is a cardiologist located in the Oak Ridge building next to Memorial Hospital."*

Obviously this discussion can be quite simple, but you will learn in time that you can reduce the length of the call if you add a disclosure about where you are located and the specialty of the practice. By adding a title to your staff member's name, such as accounts receivable manager, you will better position yourself for the next steps. Your tone of voice should be calm and friendly, and reflect a positive attitude that will set the tone for the rest of the conversation.

Step 3. Ask for payment in full

> *"Mr. Smith, our records indicate that there is a balance due on your account of $250 for a consultation that Dr. Johnson did in December. Can we expect that payment in full in the mail by this Friday, or would you like to drop it by the office today?"*

Give the patient two alternatives, both of which encourage a positive answer. Ask for payment in full even if the amount due is high. Even if

Figure 7-1: Telephone dos and don'ts

TELEPHONE DOs

1. Do know all details concerning the account.
2. Do have faith in the correctness of the account.
3. Do identify the person answering the phone.
4. Do keep calm and cheerful.
5. Do insist on a promise of payment in full.
6. Do treat all patients as you would want to be treated.
7. Do remember that everyone is right until proved otherwise.
8. Do get all the important details if the account is disputed.

TELEPHONE DON'Ts

1. Don't antagonize people.
2. Don't consider all patients "deadbeats."
3. Don't shout.
4. Don't accuse a patient of being dishonest.
5. Don't adopt a hard-boiled attitude.
6. Don't at any time threaten the patient.
7. Don't consent to small weekly payments.
8. Don't assume the full responsibility for adjusting a dispute.

your staff member feels it is unrealistic to ask for that amount, the point is that's what is owed. You can always come down, but you can't go up.

Step 4. Psychological pause

This undoubtedly is the most important step in the call. If the party doesn't respond in 10 to 12 seconds, it may seem like a lifetime to you but in essence, you have told the patient everything he or she needs to know. It's up to the patient to respond, and if you try to do it for him, you may be giving him ideas he never would have thought of independently. Therefore, no matter how long that pause lasts, wait for the response. Listening skills are very important. If the patient does not respond for a long time, ask whether he understood what you said.

Step 5. Determine the problem

> *"Miss Jones, I'm sorry, but I don't have that much money right now. I can't possibly send you $250 by Friday."*

Undoubtedly the patient will have a comment or objection. Learn what the problem is so that you can find a solution. In some cases the objection may be converted from "why I can't pay" to "why I won't pay." If you planned ahead, you should be able to answer questions right away, indicating that you know what you're talking about and have control of the situation. Listen to what the patient is saying, discover what the real problem is, and deal with it. Ask questions but don't put the patient on the defensive. You are trying to help him resolve a situation. Offer alternatives or, if necessary, suggest a payment plan that both of you can live with.

Step 6. Find the solution and close the sale

> *"Mr. Smith, we have been very reasonable and have waited long enough. You could charge it to your MasterCard or Visa."*
>
> *"I don't have any charge cards, Miss Jones."*
>
> *"Well, we expect you to send $100 by the end of the week and the balance by the end of next month. I think that is only fair, don't you."*
>
> *"Yes, Miss Jones. I will do just that."*

Try to negotiate a fair solution. Ultimately you are seeking payment in full, but be prepared to offer suggestions toward a solution. Once you get a satisfactory resolution, close the deal. This undoubtedly will be difficult for an individual with minimal experience, but keep in mind that the overall purpose of the call is to control your receivables.

Therefore, if you can't resolve the problem, you do have alternatives. For example, you can tell the patient you have no alternative but to place the account on collection. You can put the patient on a payment plan or perhaps based on their circumstances, discount the bill. Finally, remember that you will not be successful with every call, and if you try to be, the whole exercise will be uneconomical. The objective is to collect what you can as quickly as possibly and move on.

Step 7. Confirm the arrangement

> *"Mr. Smith, let me clarify what we have just discussed. You are going to send $100 to Dr. Johnson by Friday and the balance of $150 by the end of next month. Is that correct?"*

> *"Yes, it is."*

> *"Thank you, Mr. Smith. I will make a note in your file and after I receive your $100, I will send you a new statement and return envelope for next month's payment. Your address is still 2212 Harbor Street, isn't it?"*

Once you get the patient to commit to making a payment, the call doesn't stop there. Reaffirm with the patient the amount he or she is going to pay and the day when he or she is going to pay it. Be sure the patient has your correct address, and if it is an extended payment plan, ideally you should acknowledge that in writing, keeping a copy on file so there will be no misunderstanding. If you promised something, be sure to follow through. Record the outcome in the patient file, carefully noting any disputes that have arisen during the conversation.

The Second Collection Call

The most important thing to remember about collecting by telephone is that no matter how many phone calls you make, only the first two have any practical significance. The initial call is to ask for the money, and the second is to find out why the patient did not keep the promise made during the first call. If a patient makes a promise and fails to keep it, one of three things probably has occurred: (1) It was simply an oversight and the follow-up call will produce the payment; (2) immediately after the patient made a commitment for payment, the patient's circumstances dramatically changed and the patient failed to inform you that she wouldn't be able to keep the promise; or (3) the promise was made simply so that the patient could get off the phone and the patient doesn't even remember the conversation. It is important to recognize in these cases that the patient has lost face with you and that it won't be very easy for her to make another promise. The sheer fact that you're able to call the patient 10 times and get 10 promises may be an indicator that the accounts are being worked but the receivables aren't being managed.

Federal Debt Collection Practices Act

The Federal Debt Collection Practices Act (FDCPA) was adopted by Congress in the late 1970's and was designed to eliminate abusive tactics used by third party collectors. Since its enactment, a number of negative things have occurred. First, case law has led to some decisions that are not in keeping with the original intent of the act. As a result, most of the suits that are filed are based on technicalities. The FDCPA is a regulation for third party professional debt collectors, not for medical offices. However, as you will soon learn, some medical offices have crossed the line, most often by using preprinted collection dunning notices that appear to come from a third party. Therefore, examples and comments relative to this topic will give the reader an overview of the problems and challenges a collection agency may encounter and also will point out parallels to ensure that the medical office avoids being covered under the FDCPA.

The Federal Trade Commission (FTC) receives a large number of complaints yearly from consumers who believe that their rights have been violated when in fact the allegation is against the original credit granter, not a third party debt collector. As a result, under its statutory obligations to report to Congress in 1993, the FTC recommended that all credit granters be covered under the FDCPA. It is highly unlikely that if movement takes place in this area, the FTC will cover healthcare credit granters, but since legislation is unpredictable and some of the complaints have been made against hospitals, it is wise to understand what is involved.

When a consumer makes a complaint, he or she rarely indicates whether the call and/or letter came from a third party professional debt collector or an in-house collection program. In the larger medical setting, it is not uncommon for an office to have a department or individual whose sole function is to collect accounts. If that department or individual begins to sound like or look like a third party debt collection agency, the practice may have some exposure. Although those crossovers may seem inconsequential, they are consistent, and there may be so many of them that a reevaluation of the practice may be in order. Crossovers may include rephrasing "This is the office of Dr. John Doe," to "This is the credit department. We are calling about Dr. John Doe's bill." Also, giving an address different from the address normally used by Dr. John Doe could easily lead to claims by the patient that he perceived he was being contacted by a third party relative to the debt.

If a practice uses preprinted notices, the same conclusion may be reached. We list below actions that are prohibited by the FDCPA when done by a third party collection agency. I strongly encourage you to follow them so that we don't end up with federal legislation that will cover you. It is not that this act is bad; it's just that you already have enough to do. With the number of technical violations that collection agencies have encountered, you don't need the additional exposure.

Contacting Debtors

Frequency

Under the law, there is no limit on the number of times you can contact a debtor by phone. However, the law considers it a violation if the collector allows the phone to ring for a long period, or engages a debtor in conversation repeatedly or continuously to annoy or harass that person.

Time of the Day

You may contact a debtor any time between 8 a.m. and 9 p.m. local time. However, if the debtor has asked not to be contacted at a specific time, the collector may not call then. If the collector has prior consent from the debtor or permission from the court to call at other times, he or she may do so.

Where the Debtor May Be Contacted

The telephone collector may call the debtor's home or place of employment. However, if the collector knows that the debtor's employer prohibits such calls, or if the debtor has requested no calls at work, calls may not be made to the debtor at the place of employment.

Whom the Collector May Discuss the Debt With

The collector may contact the debtor, the debtor's parent, guardian, executor, administrator, or attorney when attempting to collect a debt. You may not contact relatives, friends, baby sitters, neighbors, or co-workers, unless the debtor or his or her attorney has given consent for you to do so.

Harassment of Abuse

A collector cannot engage in any conduct that harasses, oppresses or abuses any person in connection with the collection of a debt. The following acts among others are prohibited:

1. Threatening or using violence or criminal acts that might harm a person physically or affect his or her reputation or property.

2. Using obscene or profane or language that abuses the debtor.

3. Publishing a list of debtors who refuse to pay except to send to a credit reporting agency.

4. Placing telephone calls without disclosing the collector's true identity, unless engaging in skip tracing.

5. Using the telephone to annoy or harass a debtor by allowing the phone to ring continuously or calling repeatedly.

False or Misleading Representations

A collector cannot use any false, deceptive, or misleading representations to collect a debt. The following acts among others are prohibited:

1. Falsely representing yourself or implying that you are an attorney, or implying that correspondence is from an attorney.

2. Threatening to take any action that cannot be taken legally or that you have no intention of taking.

3. Falsely claiming that the debtor has committed a crime or has engaged in criminal conduct as a ploy to disgrace the debtor.

4. Falsely representing yourself as being bonded (or vouched for) by the United States or any state. This includes the use of a badge, uniform, or facsimile thereof.

5. Falsely stating that nonpayment of a debt will result in imprisonment or seizure, garnishment, or sale of any property or wages of any person unless such action is lawful and the collector or creditor intends to take such action.

6. Using false or deceptive means to collect or attempt to collect a debt or obtain information about a debtor.

7. Falsely representing or implying that documents given to a debtor are legal and were filed under due process.

8. Falsely representing the character, amount, or legal status of a debt or any services rendered or compensation which may be lawfully received by a collector for the collection of a debt.

9. Communicating or threatening to communicate credit information which is or should be known to be false, including failure to communicate the fact that a disputed debt is in fact disputed.

10. Falsely representing or implying that if any interest in the debt is sold, referred, or transferred, such action may cause the debtor to lose the claim or defense to payment of the debt.

11. Using any business, organization, or company name other than the true name of the entity attempting to collect a debt. Such an action

automatically places the collector in violation of the FTC Code and the Federal Consumer Protection Act.

12. Except as provided under the skip tracing section of the law, failing to clearly disclose in all communications intended to collect a debt or obtain information about a consumer (other than location information) that the collector is attempting to collect a debt and that this information will be used for that purpose.

Unfair Practices

Again, the following list is for collection agencies, not medical practices. Nevertheless, some practices add an additional charge to an account when it is transferred to a collection agency with the thought that the additional charge will cover the contingency fee. However, under FDCPA, this is considered an unfair practice. Thus, you cannot do the following:

1. Collect any amount (including interest, fee, charge, or expense incidental to the principal obligation) unless that amount is expressly authorized by the agreement creating the debt or is permitted by law.

2. Communicate with a debtor about a debt by postcard. This violates the debtor's privacy.

3. Accept from any person a check or other payment instrument that is postdated by more than five days unless that person is notified in writing of the collector's intention to deposit the check not more than 10 or less than three business days before making the deposit.

4. Depositing or threatening to deposit any postdated check or other payment instrument before the date of the check.

5. Soliciting a postdated check or another payment instrument for the purpose of threatening or initiating criminal proceedings.

6. Taking or threatening to take any nonjudicial action to dispossess or disable property if there is no right to possession of the property claimed as collateral through an enforceable security interest, if there is no intention to take possession of the property, or if the property is exempt by law from such action.

The Medical Office And The FDCPA

Most medical offices conduct themselves within the parameters of the FDCPA. However, there are a few common practices of medical offices that may be in violation of the FDCPA. Several companies sell preprinted collection letters to healthcare facilities that imply to the

Figure 7-2: Notices for collection agencies required by the FDCPA

VALIDATION NOTICE

Required on the Collection Agency's First Statement

Unless you notify this office in writing within 30 days from receiving this notice that you dispute the validity of the debt or any portion thereof, this office will assume this debt is valid. If you notify this office in writing within 30 days from receiving this notice, this office will obtain verification of the debt or obtain a copy of the judgement and mail you a copy of such judgement or notification.

DISCLOSURE STATEMENT

Required on Every Written Communication by the Collection Agency

This is an attempt to collect a debt. Any information obtained will be used for that purpose.

---

patient that the letter is coming from a collection agency. This is a violation of FDCPA because it constitutes deceptive practice. Some medical offices' final notices could be construed as duns, and it is possible to argue that these offices are in violation because the notice failed to provide the validation notice, which is a lengthy paragraph giving the debtor the right to dispute the bill and a second written notification that the purpose of the communication is to collect a debt and that any information obtained will be used for that purpose. These notices, which must be used by collection agencies in written communication, are shown in Figure 7-2.

I am not suggesting that a healthcare provider needs to use these two notices, but you must recognize that an overly aggressive program of A/R management can be viewed as a violation of the act. This is especially true if your employee calls patients and states that he or she is with the XYZ Collection Agency rather than with your office.

The Consequences Of FDCPA Violations Or Allegations Of Violations

Since you are probably beginning to wonder why I am stressing the FDCPA when it doesn't pertain to you, I would like to share two incidents that happened recently. Although to the best of my knowledge both cases occurred with third party medical billers, the same scenarios could apply to a medical practice which does its own billing. There are several things you need to keep in mind. First, FDCPA is a federal law and therefore, any alleged violation of it is tried in a federal court. It is generally felt that the cost of defending oneself in a federal court can run $4,000 to $6,000. Second, the statutory fine for the violation plus attorney fees if you are found guilty can easily add up to several thousand dollars. In addition, very few third party medical collectors and/or medical practices have errors and omissions insurance, which can help defray these expenses if there is such an allegation.

When allegations of violations of the FDCPA are made against third party debt collectors, it is not uncommon for the attorney to be willing to settle out of court for a significantly lesser sum. In addition, if the allegation is tried in court, it is done so with the consumer being viewed as "the least sophisticated," which in essence means that no matter how logical the process was, if it can be determined that the consumer could have perceived it in another manner, then that's the way it is.

Scenario One

In the first scenario, a patient received a statement which at the very top said "past due" in large letters. The body of the letter alleged that the practice was going to take legal action, which it had never done before. At the bottom of the letter was the physician's name and address of record. The allegations were plentiful. The first allegation was that the consumer concluded that he had received a notice which he perceived was from a third-party debt collector. If that point had been established, the allegations that followed would include the fact that the party sending the letter should have been covered under the FDCPA and failed to include the validation and disclosure notices required under the law. The notice was sent in one of 29 states which require state licensing; since this organization was not licensed, a violation occurred. The third allegation said that the action threatened in the letter was a deceptive practice since the credit granter never had taken such an action in the past. In this scenario and the one to follow, both individuals made a business decision to settle out of court.

Scenario Two

In the second scenario, an initial statement itemizing all the services rendered was mailed to a patient informing him that insurance had been filed. Shortly thereafter, the insurance company paid and another statement was mailed stating that this balance was his responsibility. Then, a month or so later, a third statement went out stating that the balance was delinquent and that the patient had to remit immediately to the credit department. Unfortunately, the patient had died. Nevertheless, an allegation was made that the statement inferred a third party collection agency and lacked the required disclosures. Even though in all probability the defendant would have prevailed, the amount at risk was too great, and an out-of-court settlement was made.

Again, none of this is intended to be a scare tactic. However, if you're sending a final notice on canary yellow paper with large block red printing, that might suggest that it came from a third party.

Credit Bureaus And Their Use By Medical Offices

In many areas of the country, credit bureaus accept negative information on the medical accounts of patients who don't pay. On the surface this may sound like a wonderful idea. However, I do not recommend it unless you have an incredibly large volume of past-due accounts and an in-house collection staff that is going to continue to work those accounts. The major reason I do not encourage reporting to a credit bureau is that if you list it with the bureau and the patient pays, you need to reverse the information and remove it from the bureau's records. This usually can be done with a phone call or letter, but because of high turnover or a constantly changing system, the probability of ineffective updating of credit information by a busy medical office is high.

The second reason I hesitate to recommend using credit bureau reporting as a means of controlling A/R is that negative information in a credit bureau report comes to the debtor's attention only when he or she attempts to secure additional credit. Most likely a person will not know if indebtedness to a physician, a hospital or another medical facility is on his or her credit bureau report unless he or she tries to obtain a home equity loan, buy a new home or car, or refinance an existing home. A delinquency of this nature needs to be worked by a collection agency, rather than being treated as a one-time remedy. Collection agencies are set up to handle mass reporting and eradicating of credit bureau information.

Reverse Directories And Skip Tracing

Collection agencies have several other tools. One of the most useful is known as a reverse directory or crisscross directory. A reverse directory basically lists every address in a city along with the name and phone number, if available, of the individual who lives there. Some directories even list how long a party has lived at an address. It is a wonderful device if you get a mail return and run into a dead end trying to locate a patient. By checking the last known address of the patient in the directory, you can often locate a neighbor of that patient and call that person, asking where you might locate the patient. Quite often a neighbor will know.

There is a skip tracing service that involves a computer bulletin board system and is available to collection agencies. It is a huge database, and for a fee, a collection agency can hook up to that database and search through records, usually by using a Social Security number, to find a person who has "skipped" out on an account. This system is not readily available to medical offices directly, but many collection agencies should soon be able to hook up to the system.

Both of these collection tools are not feasible choices for the vast majority of medical offices, mainly because of their cost in comparison with the amount they will return. Moreover, if you take all the other steps recommended in this book, you probably won't have the time or manpower to use them. If you do, you've gone beyond the scope of basic management of you're a/R and are acting like a third party collector.

Summary

The telephone is an effective device for controlling you're a/R when it is used in an appropriate fashion. It should not, however, be the primary method for controlling receivables because it is labor-intensive. Most importantly it should be recognized that repeated and multiple calls to the same patient defeat the overall goal of managing your receivables. However, when the telephone is used, this should be done by an individual who has been trained to use it effectively and efficiently.

Some of the most important aspects of effective telephone collection practices are goal setting, proper planning, maintaining a positive attitude, keeping control of the situation, listening to what the patient is saying, and negotiating and closing the "deal." The collection industry has established a seven-step system for making a successful collection phone call, which may be helpful to a practice in managing its receivables. The seven steps are as follows: (1) identify the party, (2) identify yourself, (3) ask for payment in full, (4) pause and wait for a response, (5) learn the problem, (6) find a solution and close the deal, and (7) confirm the arrangement. If the first phone call is done properly, a second one should be unnecessary.

Although it does not directly pertain to a medical practice, the Fair Debt Collection Practices Act is a federal law of which a practice should be aware. There have been a few cases in recent years where billing offices were scrutinized for deceptive practices because these looked and acted like collection agencies. Credit bureau reporting and skip tracing mechanisms are another aspect of the collection industry that should be avoided because of their cost.

The individuals in a medical practice who are given the responsibility of making patient contacts for the purpose of collecting should be supported by all staff members, particularly the principals of the practice, in regard to the payment policies that have been established. Both mechanically and philosophically, the members of the practice have to work in concert to ensure that the telephone will be an effective tool.

CHAPTER 8

DELINQUENCY: ITS CAUSES AND REMEDIES

When a practitioner renders a service to a patient and is not immediately paid for that service, he or she becomes a credit granter, although an unwilling one. If, for example, the fee for an office visit is $50, any patient who does not pay on the day of service has been "lent" that amount. Something of value was provided to the patient, and no compensation was made. Physicians in a hospital-based practice extend credit to all their patients. Practices that request payment at time of service may not grant as much credit but still are credit granters for some patients.

By being a credit granter, you are in competition with other credit granters for your debtor's dollars, since nearly every person in the United States owes money to someone for something. You hope the patient will pay in full after they receive the first statement, but if the bill isn't paid after several months, it becomes delinquent. This chapter will help a practitioner understand how debtors become delinquent and get a head start in collecting some of the credit that has been extended to your patients.

Psychology 101: The Concept Of Needs

Many courses in business psychology include a discussion of psychologist Abraham Maslow's theory of human motivation. Maslow's theory states that all people have an internal need structure that begins with the basic for food and shelter and moves upward until it reaches the ultimate level of self-fulfillment. However, before one can achieve the higher needs, the needs at all the lower levels must be met. Also, some needs are satisfied only to reappear again, such as physical needs. By keeping these needs in mind while discussing delinquency with a patient, one can direct an appeal to a number of need levels at the same time. Those need levels, from lowest to highest, are physical, psychological, social, ego and self-fulfillment.

Level 1. Physical

Physical needs are things that are necessary for existence, including food, water, shelter, health, and sleep. A person cannot concentrate on any needs higher on the ladder until these basic needs are satisfied.

Patients who are worried about physical needs are difficult to motivate to make payment in full.

Level 2. Psychological

Psychological needs are things that satisfy the feelings of security and safety. Some people set aside a nest egg for emergencies and do not want to part with that form of security. Others are uncertain about a job and don't want to make any commitments they cannot meet. Motivating a person who is lacking security to pay a medical bill requires thoughtful coercing.

Level 3. Social

At the point where an individual is physically comfortable and has minimal fear for safety, the social needs have primary influence on his behavior. These are the needs of belonging, being loved and maintaining friendships. An appeal to his honesty and stature in the community can sometimes motivate him into payment.

Level 4. Ego

Ego needs are needs that relate to an individual's self-esteem and reputation. They also include the needs for self-confidence, recognition, appreciation and respect. Patients in this category are often embarrassed about owing money. Often, their medical indebtedness may be due to serious illness or catastrophic event, and they are frustrated by their inability to pay. Patience and understanding are required in the listener.

Level 5. Self Fulfillment

When all other needs have been satisfied, such as the needs for creativity and continued development, the individual seeks the things that are ultimately self-fulfilling. These people are interested in themselves and don't want anything to get in their way. An appeal for payment so that they don't have to worry about the debt again may be appropriate.

Consumer Credit Attitudes

Fortunately, most people want to pay their bills. Unfortunately, sometimes they don't have the resources to pay all their debts and must decide which ones to pay first. Remember that a patient who owes you money probably needs to pay for food and shelter and most likely uses retail credit. You are in competition for a patient's credit dollar. Even though everyone in the medical profession knows that medical debts are as genuine as retail debts, some patients just don't feel the same

Figure 8-1: Priority list of average consumer's bill paying

1. Mortgage or rent payment

2. Car payment

3. Telephone and other utilities

4. Bank loan

5. Furniture and appliance installments

6. Credit card account

7. Insurance premiums

8. Medical, dental, and hospital bills

obligation. Motivation for payment varies from individual to individual. People tend to pay first for obligations that were obtained by choice and represent personal comfort. Market research on consumer credit shows that the average person decides to pay their bills in the order as shown in Figure 8-1.

These categories include only the average consumer's regular bills. If you consider that people still have to buy food and clothing, medicine, and personal products, it is not surprising that medical bills sink ever lower on the list of bills to pay. Because people prioritize their bill paying in this way, the most recent figures indicate that losses on credit extended by people in the medical field is two to three times those of people who grant retail credit.

Debtors' reasons for not paying range from extreme financial difficulties to a refusal to pay. As described in Chapter 5, a firm credit policy not only is desirable but in some cases is totally necessary. Chapter 3 stressed the importance of each financial class, especially self-pay, have a billing cycle that is tailored to meet its criteria. A medical office must put the care of the patient above all else but should communicate clearly to the patient exactly what his or her financial obligation is and the moral responsibility to pay it.

Causes Of Delinquency

Even though most people want to pay their bills in a timely manner, sometimes they simply cannot for a host of reasons. Sometimes medical expenses are unexpected and funds were not set aside for the unplanned obligation. For whatever reason, some people become delinquent in paying their bills. With a clear understanding of the general reasons behind a debtor's delinquency, a medical office can tailor its approach to achieve a successful outcome. Generally, delinquencies are attributed to one of four categories: circumstantial, intellectual, emotional and intentional.

Circumstantial Causes

Many individuals are in debt because of circumstances they cannot anticipate or control: natural disasters, unemployment, sickness, sudden death, or a personal injury. Anyone can fall into this category at one time or another. The majority of these individuals are seeking a way to get out of debt, but in many cases there is no light at the end of the tunnel. Somehow they failed to communicate with the credit granter to try to work out a solution.

Intellectual Causes

Many adults are not capable of budgeting their income. They do not plan ahead and have difficulty keeping elementary financial records. Very often they have no idea about how much money they will have after meeting their basic expenses. These debtors usually want to pay but need lessons in handling their financial affairs. With the help of a credit counseling service, many of them eventually pay their bills and get started on a path to solvency.

Emotional Causes

This is a relatively small group of individuals think the world owes them something, and make purchases without knowing how they are going to pay for them. Often they find themselves overextended. Unlike mature adults who face the situation and make arrangements with their creditors, emotionally immature people often try to bluff their way through the situation. Debt caused by emotional causes is by far the most difficult to deal with because it normally involves individuals who simply don't care. When immature debtors are pressured to pay, they become anxious and fearful and try to defend themselves from real and imagined consequences by using tactics such as lying, stalling, and running. If you can penetrate these defenses and learn the true state of affairs, you often can persuade this type of person to pay.

Intentional Causes

People who intentionally use fraud and deception to receive goods and services with no intention of ever paying for them are true credit criminals. They will use any excuse not to pay their bills. Sometimes they write bad checks, and they are often the "skips" mentioned in earlier chapters. These types of debtors are the most irritating and the hardest to deal with.

Classifying A Debtor By Anticipated Results

Once a debt becomes delinquent, it is usually referred to a collection agency. Professional debt collectors have the ability to categorize debtors on the basis of the expected results of the collection effort. This system can help increase your success rate as well. For the most part, patients who are delinquent in paying a bill fit into one or more of these groups. They reveal their classification as soon as they tell you why they haven't paid. Once they have been classified, patient-debtors help you choose the best collection approach.

The Patient Who Is Willing to Make Arrangements to Satisfy the Debt

As was stated earlier, most people want to pay their debts. They are in financial trouble for a reason which is beyond their control. Through careful negotiation, a payment plan can be arranged which will be satisfactory for both parties. Included in this classification are the following:

1. **Victims of adverse circumstances:** These people customarily pay their bills promptly but are temporarily unable to do so. Circumstances beyond their control, such as illness or loss of employment, have put them in a difficult financial position. People who owe large medical bills but lack adequate insurance also fall into this category.

2. **Poor budgeter:** Some people go through life nonchalantly and buy almost anything on credit. These people seldom budget and tend to live in the present rather than plan for the future. They often make purchases that reflect desire instead of need. Many chronic debtors fall into this category, which is often characterized by people who are unable or unwilling to accept responsibility for managing their own affairs.

3. **Those with limited income or large families:** These circumstances can make keeping up with bill paying a difficult task. However, these debtors are usually willing to try to find a solution.

The Debtor with a Grievance or Dispute

Many debtors offer the excuse that they were unhappy with the service they received or had a dispute of some nature. You must learn to discriminate between a legitimate grievance and a stall. The chances are great that the alibi is a stall. Listen for a tone of sincerity but do put the burden of proof on the debtor. If it sounds like a valid dispute, check it out immediately and do what you can to resolve the matter. Urgency is the key here, because the longer the dispute lingers, the more the patient becomes convinced that he or she is right.

The Staller

The staller gives every reason for putting off paying the account. These excuses range from "one more week," to an imaginary dispute, to demands for itemized statements or a schedule of small payments. In dealing with this type of debtor, you must use a sense of urgency in asking for payment.

The Debtor Who Refuses to Pay But Can Be Motivated

These debtors are forthright about not paying and often embellish their refusal with a bit of profanity. Either they are bluffing or they believe you will not or cannot take steps to force payment. If your best collection efforts fail to convince them, you will have to resort to legal action.

The Debtor Who Refuses to Pay and Cannot Be Motivated

This type falls into three classes: credit criminals, skips, and hardship cases.

1. **Credit Criminals**. These debtors obtain credit whenever and wherever they can. They move frequently and often use variations of their given names to throw creditors off the track. A careful search usually reveals that they have no assets. Most creditors close their files on this type of account, report it to a credit reporting agency, and place the account in the inactive file for periodic review.

2. **Skips**. Although credit criminals leaves town for fraudulent reasons, not all skips are deliberately evading their creditors. Some have moved and in the turmoil of leaving have forgotten to give a forwarding address to the post office. Sometimes a skip begins in this innocent manner, but as time goes by and nothing happens, he or she becomes less inclined to consider the debt an obligation. In dealing with a skip, consider the action as an innocent oversight until you have reason to believe otherwise.

3. **Hardship cases**. In a true case of hardship, where the debtor is physically or mentally handicapped or destitute, there probably is no question about honesty. The debtor is simply unable to earn enough to pay the bill. Most creditors charge off this type of account. This file belongs in your closed accounts. Keep in mind, however, that only a small percentage of accounts should fall into this category.

It is good to understand the types of debtors you may be confronted with. This will give you a better perspective on how to handle their complaints and problems and eventually reach the goal of payment in full (PIF).

What To Do When An Account Becomes Delinquent

You've been mailing statements religiously for 4 or 5 months. Nothing. You have sent a very professional and appealing personal collection letter. Nothing. You have had your staff try to contact the patient by telephone. Nothing. Enough is enough. It is time to take action.

In-House Efforts

When an account becomes delinquent, the first thing that probably comes to mind is intensified efforts by your staff. You form an in-house collection team. One or more staff members are assigned the task of calling and writing the delinquent patient's repeatedly. Seemingly, this is an inexpensive way to handle delinquent patients because you are not paying fees to an outside firm. However, in the long run this method can be quite costly. Remember the black hole and the seven percent rule. Consider the salaries of the individuals who are working these accounts. You are using your staff members' time to work on accounts at the back end of your receivables, and this takes valuable time away from the more collectible accounts at the front end of your receivables. This is not a very effective way to manage A/R.

Precollection Services

Instead of intensifying collection efforts in the office when an account becomes delinquent, an alternatives is to use outside agencies, or "outsourcing" for precollection services. Many collection agencies offer this type of service, which is especially attractive for a practice that has a big A/R problem and insufficient staff to handle it. Precollection services can be provided in a number of ways for a reasonable cost. One method is to have the collection agency send the final notice on their letterhead instead of yours. The letter will usually state that the agency has been retained by you to secure payment before the account goes into its regular collection cycle. It gives the patient a last chance to pay before the account goes to collection. The letter can direct payments and inquiries either to the physician's office or to the outsource. The letter has a much greater impact than does your final notice because of the presence of a third party. In addition, some collection agencies that offer this service send a follow-up letter or make a phone call before turning the account over for collection.

A simple precollect letter is shown in Figure 8-2. Note that the agency has included a disclaimer clause. This is a requirement under the Federal Debt Collection Practices Act, which governs collection agencies (Chapter 7).

Figure 8-2: Sample precollection letter

XYZ COLLECTION SERVICES
1234 Main Street
Anywhere, U.S.A. 11111
(555) 555-5555

Date

John Doe
4321 Elm St.
Anywhere, U.S.A. 11111

RE: Mary Strangelove, M.D. Account #12345, Balance Due $120.00

Dear Mr. Doe:

XYZ Collection Services has been retained by Dr. Mary Strangelove in reference to a balance of $120.00 past due on account 12345 for professional services rendered.

We have been asked by the physician to resolve this matter within the next 30 days so the account need not go to collection. Therefore, your prompt response will be appreciated. Please send your payment to:

XYZ Collection Services
1234 Main Street
Anywhere, U.S.A. 11111

or call (555) 555-5555

This is an attempt to collect a debt. Any information obtained will be used for that purpose.

Unless you notify this office in writing within 30 days of receiving this notice that you dispute the validity of the debt or any portion thereof, this office will assume this debt is valid. If you notify this office in writing within 30 days of receiving this notice, this office will obtain verification of the debt or obtain a copy of the judgment and mail you a copy of such judgment or notification.

Sincerely,

Collection Agent

Charges for precollect services can be as a flat rate per account, letter, or phone call; a small contingency fee; or a combination of the two. Of course, this is a negotiable item between a practice and an agency. After a predetermined period, usually 30 days or less, these accounts are turned over to the agency for its regular collection services.

Professional Collection Agency

When a self-pay account becomes delinquent, the most efficient thing to do is refer it to a collection agency for full collection services. The criteria for sending an account to a collection agency don't necessarily relate to a time frame. If the patient has repeatedly promised payment and has not followed through, the account should go to collection. If you have lost contact with the patient because of an incorrect address or because the patient has moved away, it is time to try the efforts of a professional collector. If the patient has a personal problem such as unemployment or has refused to pay, the account should be referred to a collection agency. Collectors are professionals. This is what they do, and they do it for a fee that is not only fair but well spent. Chapter 10 covers the selection and monitoring of a professional collection agency.

Attorneys

In some instances it may be desirable to refer an account directly to an attorney for proceedings. Sometimes a collection agency will, with the permission of the practitioner, request legal action on an account. This generally occurs where recovery is possible and the cost can be justified, such as a large balance of several thousand dollars and documentation that the patient received reimbursement from an insurance company. In cases like these, an account can be referred directly to a law firm that specializes in debt collection. This has an impact because it informs the patient that you are serious about recovering the money owed to you. The downside is that it is usually very costly and the attorney will often ask for up-front costs. In addition, it can take months or years before a settlement is reached and you receive payment.

Small Claims Court

You can sue a patient in small claims court even for a relatively small amount. The obvious advantage, as with referring to an attorney, is the strong impact it will have in conveying your serious intentions. If you win the case, which in all likelihood you will, you can garnish debtor's wages or have a lien put on their property. Unfortunately, a judgement does not necessary mean you will be paid. It can stay on a debtor's record for years as long as the debtor does not sell a house or apply for an equity loan. In addition, the process is very time consuming and you may have to pay court costs.

Write-Offs

In many cases it is fruitless to pursue certain accounts beyond a certain point. Accounts in this category include small balances, a death with no estate, and destitute patients. The best thing you can do is write off the account. If you have the type of billing system that keeps on billing these accounts, you are wasting money. Also, your will have an inflated A/R if you keep these accounts on your books. Don't hang on to them any longer. Save time and money by writing them off.

Summary

Voluntarily or involuntarily, when you provide a service to a patient and agree to bill the patient foe the service, you become a credit granter. If you bill the patient in a timely manner and the patient does not pay promptly, he or she becomes a delinquent debtor. You cannot control the patient's reason for owing money to your practice, but you can make your practice more efficient by weeding out marginal accounts as quickly as possible. In working with delinquent patients, it is important to remember that the vast majority are looking for a solution; in some cases that may mean a reasonable payment plan or a significant discount in the amount of the debt. It is also important to understand that not every debt can be collected.

Although it is not always easy to classify why a patient owes you money, each type of debtor is going to respond differently to different types of appeals. A philosopher once said that if the only tool in your toolbox is a hammer, you will treat everything as if it were a nail. Therefore, the better you do the job of classifying delinquencies, the more tactful you can be in finding the most effective tool to get the highest recovery of you're a/R dollar.

CHAPTER 9

CONTROLLING YOUR CONTRACTUAL RELATIONSHIPS

It would be nice if all the contractual relationships in a medical practice were consciously and willingly created. It would even be nicer if third parties could not interfere in the financial relationship between a practitioner and a patient. That isn't the way it works. Today a physician has to deal with federally run programs such as Medicare, state-structured plans like Medicaid, insurance companies with a concept of "usual and customary" fees, contractual managed care programs that call for discounts and carve-outs (those specific procedures excluded from the contract that will not be discounted) and non-contractual programs to which everyone but the physician agreed.

As a result, most patients today have a third party intervening, sometimes dictating what the compensation will be for the services that were rendered and the timeliness of that compensation. More and more staff time is needed for managing A/R and meeting the specific needs of those third party interventions. This chapter describes the defensive and offensive steps a practice can take and gives a few pointers that should be considered before you sign a managed care contract.

It would be difficult to determine exactly when the old philosophy of physician's compensation ceased to exist: Patient sees doctor, doctor treats patient, and then the financial details are worked out. The current philosophy seems to be "Doctor, if you treat this patient for this ailment, this is the very maximum you will receive, and no telling when." This sounds cynical, but I work in a business that deals with the aftermath of misunderstandings. I am convinced that it is the practitioner who is taking most of the mistreatment, not the patient or the third party that controls the coverage. Therefore, this chapter is biased in favor of all the people who provide healthcare. A handful of these individuals may have helped create the problem, but the pendulum has swung too far against medical practitioners.

Let us look at the many aspects of insurance reimbursement and managed care and examine how they affect the management of A/R. Rather than attempting to determine when and where the problem started, let us look at some of the definitions that are currently used, where they came from, what their original intention was, and what they mean now.

Usual, Customary, Reasonable Reimbursement

The usual, customary, reasonable (UCR) form of reimbursement was originally intended to mean the following:

Usual: what most doctors usually charge. The original definition went a step further by referring to what most doctors usually charge in a geographic area. This has caused the term to have regional differences.

Customary: what a particular physician has customarily charged over a period of time. Obviously, the longer the time period is the lower that amount will be.

Reasonable: what the payer feels is reasonable. This term also makes this situation highly subjective.

Very often this terminology is referred to simply as usual and customary (U&C). This was the definition which came into play in the mid-1980s, when Medicare recognized that it had to put some restraints on what it paid for. However, beginning with a very large worker's compensation insurer, in the middle and late 1980s practitioners began to receive insurance checks for less than what had been charged. With these checks came an explanation of benefits (EOB), which contained a statement to the effect that the insurance company had found the charge to be higher than the U&C of other physicians in the same area. Somehow it reached the point where the patients were asked to contact their insurance carrier if the provider of care attempted to collect more than what had been determined to be the U&C. In some cases the payer offered to help defray the court costs of defending a patient against a suit for payment.

The problems in the field of healthcare reimbursement have become almost inconceivable. During the first attempt by the Clinton administration to change healthcare reimbursement in the United States, more Americans became to believe that physicians were overcharging. Any rational appeal to a patient with an outstanding balance was useless because of confirmation by the media that physicians were overcharging.

The Importance of Having an Adequate Database

When the term of "usual, customary and reasonable" was originally defined by Medicare, Medicare did have a large database and could establish a U&C by a given discipline in a given geographic area. However, there were some glitches including one I'll never forget.

On the south side of Chicago, near Cook County Hospital, there was an older practitioner who practiced in the field of internal medicine. As a result of his standing in the community, the great need for his services in his geographic area, and the fact that he practiced 7 days a week, he saw an incredible number of patients. At the same time he never modified the fee schedule he had set up in the late 1950s. His statistical contribution to the Medicare files was so substantial that even when it was combined with that of all the other internal medicine practitioners in geographic area 16, principally Cook County, he dragged down the U&C fee by an incredible percentage. As a result, in this case it was rational and reasonable for other practitioners to argue that the UCR for this geographic area was inappropriate. However, for the most part, the system of UCR worked quite well by specialty.

Although there were always inequities in that system, Medicare did in fact create a database that could create a norm. Unfortunately, when other third party payers started to use the same thinking, their databases for determining U&C were very limited and could not compare to Medicare's database. Some carriers received data from a national institute. Many others attempted to create data on the basis of the claims they received. In many cases the geographic norms changed dramatically. A disastrous situation occurred every time the statistics from a rural area were combined with those from an urban area, as this automatically dragged the U&C. More important, many of these databases were running 2 to 4 years behind the actual charge levied by practitioners.

U&C Determined by Carrier Alone

A policyholder has no way of knowing in advance or controlling what the insurance company believes is a U&C charge. Thus, his or her coverage is only as good as what the insurance company deems necessary and reasonable. Insurance companies have modified many of their form letters regarding U&C so that they now read, "If the practitioner can give us a rationale as to why your care would require this additional cost, we will be happy to consider it." Realistically, what can a practitioner say that was not on the original claim form? The problem is worsened by the fact that as these claims are paid at well below the normal value, they are added to the database of the insurance company as usual and customary. What ultimately happens is that the U&C keeps dropping because as each physician's charges are discounted, the insurance company looks at the discounted amount as the U&C. It becomes a vicious cycle.

Defenses and Offenses To Ensure Payment of the Full Amount

The real problem with the concept of U&C can be seen in cases where an insurance company disallows portions of a physician's charges even though the physician has no contractual relationship with that company. A patient is responsible for the full charge, yet the insurance company tells the patient that the physician has overcharged. Let's look at a simple scenario and use it to talk about the offenses and defenses that should be in place.

Let's look at a situation taking place in an office-based setting, although some of these principles also apply to hospital-based practitioners. A patient calls the practitioner's office and makes an appointment. She comes in and receives the appropriate treatment. At the conclusion of that treatment, she is given a bill and is told as a courtesy that a claim will be filed with her insurance company. The practitioner's office files the insurance claim, having benefits assigned to the practitioner. Shortly afterward, a check is received at the practitioner's office with an EOB attached. Clearly printed on the EOB is a statement by the carrier saying that after careful review that it finds that the charge should have been substantially less, and as a result it is paying only a certain amount of dollars.

The problem at this point is not economic reimbursement but public relations. The EOB from the carrier has instilled a distrust between a physician and patient by insinuating that the physician has overcharged. After all the hoopla about healthcare reform in the early 1990s, it is more than likely that the patient is going to side with the insurance company. What are your defenses?

Defense 1. Advise Patient in Advance of the Probable Charge and the Responsibility to Pay

When the patient called to make the initial appointment, it should have been explained then the practice has fixed fees for the services and the patient should have been told what the charges would be. Explain that the physician's office staff will be happy to complete any insurance claim forms, but only as a courtesy, since there is no contractual relationship between the physician and the insurance company and the physician did not participate in the selection of the patient's insurance.

Defense 2. Have Patient Sign a Patient Understanding Agreement

Since defense 1 is a lot to get out during an initial appointment, try defense 2. When a patient arrives for the first appointment, ask the patient to complete a patient information form, as was discussed in previous chapters. There can be a space on the form where a patient signs an agreement stating that he or she understand that he or she will be charged for the service at the prevailing rate charged by this practice. Explain that the patient is responsible for 100 percent of that fee regardless of what the insurance pays. This is very similar to what the major credit card companies are doing: When a person signs a charge ticket, that person is signing an agreement stating that he or she is responsible for that amount, whether or not he or she pays the credit card company. This patient understanding agreement can be expanded to point out that there are instances when insurance companies pay less than the normal fee and that some pay the entire amount. Since the practitioner did not negotiate the insurance the entire fee will be due regardless of any actions taken by the insurance company.

Figure 9-1: Sample usual and customary letter

John R. Doe, M.D.
1234 Main Street
Anywhere, U.S.A. 11111

Date

Dear Patient,

It is important to understand that you, not I, selected the insurance coverage for you and your family. As a result, neither I nor anyone on my staff participated in the review as to what medical benefits you would receive for this procedure. Therefore, any discrepancy between my charges and what your insurance carrier pays is between you and your insurance carrier.

The fact that your insurance company has told you that my charges are above what is considered usual and customary is something you need to resolve with them because the fees that I charge are similar to those of other practitioners in the same speciality and in this immediate area. You may find that your carrier is using information that is several years old or information that encompasses a broad geographic area.

In any case, we do expect payment in full for these services.

Sincerely,

Dr. John Doe

cc: Your Insurance Carrier

Offense 1. Challenge the U&C Fee

Every practice should have a form letter to send when it receives an EOB from an insurance company stating that the fee was in excess of what is considered usual and customary. Figure 9-1 shows a form letter addressed to a patient that puts the responsibility back in the patient's lap, with a copy sent to the insurance carrier. A letter to the insurance company could challenge it on the data it used to determine the U&C for those services. This is also a good policy to state to carriers that pay in full: a copy of the letter will also go to the patient, and this will help in dealing with public relations. The letter could even challenge the insurance company to submit the dispute to arbitration at the local county medical society if you feel that your fees are in line.

Offense 2. If There Is No Response, Appeal to The Insurance Commissioner

If the insurance company does not respond to the letter within 30 days, consideration should be given to sending a letter to the state insurance commissioner explaining that you have received a remittance that you feel is inappropriate, that you wrote to the carrier, and that the carrier failed to respond within an appropriate time frame.

Just Do Something

I recognize that each of these steps requires additional staff time and cost to execute, but unless physicians individually and collectively challenge carriers, distrust between patients and practitioners will continue to build. Another issue that has come out of this whole situation is the legality of accepting a check for less than what was billed and was believed to be unacceptable by the practitioner. I know of situations in which patients have challenged practitioners by stating that once the check was accepted, a contractual relationship was established. A way to avoid this confrontation is to use an endorsement stamp that says that the payment was "accepted in protest as partial payment of the obligation due." In essence, what I am suggesting is that you do something. Simply accepting the partial payment and then having the account move on to collection only reinforces the possibility that the charge was excessive in the first place. If you are wondering why I suggest such strong alternatives for a $5 or $6 differential, let me assure you that in the majority of cases with which I deal, payments have sunk to a fifth of the physicians's charge. If one is looking for a bright spot, that's it. The discrepancies have become so large that even the patient knows that something is wrong.

Fee-Based Reimbursement

The method of reimbursement known as fee-based is one in which the payer pays a percentage of the physician's actual fee, typically 80 percent of the amount charged on the claim. This method was the basis for most insurance policies in the 1960s and early 1970s. However, as payers looked for ways to reduce their exposure, many of their policies, even though still involving a fee-based method of reimbursement, added the criteria of UCR. Therefore, in recent years many beneficiaries have been covered under policies that ultimately end up paying 80 percent of the UCR, which simply increases the go between what the provider charged and what the insurance paid. Although fee-based reimbursement is not significantly different from the standard U&C type of payment, it provides an amount that is smaller, since it is only 80 percent of the U&C. The defenses and offenses outlined above are appropriate in this environment. It points to the need for a practice to get confirmation from patients that they understand that they are responsible for the full charges, not for what the insurance pays or says is reasonable.

Relative Value Systems And Their Development

In the mid-1950s practitioners saw the need for an objective method for establishing fees. What was needed was a system that used standardized nomenclature in the form of a coding system that was specific enough to cover practitioners across the country who perform the same service. As a result, the California Relative Value System (CRVS) was published. A relative value fee is based on the resources needed to perform a specific procedure, including the physician's time and skill, the experience required, the severity of the illness, and the amount of risk involved. One of the earliest examples of this occurred in the field of anesthesia, which took this concept and assigned units for every CPT code, along with units for time and other criteria. This sum was then multiplied by the practitioner's conversion factor. For example, if the total relative value units totaled 11 and the physician said that his or her conversion factor was $55 per unit, consistency of the fees charged could be maintained. The only arguable aspect of this occurred when the doctor's conversion factor was perceived to be higher than the norm.

The initial system allotted a relative value for each identifiable procedure. For the practitioner to determine the appropriate fee, he or she simply multiplied the relative value units by a conversion factor, a fixed dollar amount that varied with the type of discipline. Although this method was later tested in federal court, it became not only an objective method but one that allowed easy communication with the patient about the probable cost of service. However, for this system to function objectively, every medical procedure must be linked to a number and assigned to a level of reimbursement. The system includes the assumption that a practitioner will treat a patient only in a specific way under a code. For example, when a patient is undergoing a physical exam, and in the process carries on a non-medical dialogue with the practitioner, to justify the extra time spent, the only recourse for the physician is to charge for an extended visit and use the corresponding CPT code for such a visit. It is unfortunate that a practitioner must classify time spent with patients under CPT code when patients look to the physician as a dispenser of cures.

Relative value systems and some sort of coding will continue to be facts of life in the healthcare field. Since their inception, these systems have evolved into three types of systems: consensus systems, fee-based systems, and resource-based systems. This is how insurance carriers determine whether fees are UCR.

Consensus-based Relative Value Systems

The consensus system uses all the original tenants of the original relative value systems (RVS), which include risk, time, and procedure. Basically, it polls selected providers to determine the difficulty level of procedures. It also assesses the risk factor involved in each procedure. Furthermore, it gets a consensus of the normal amount of time and level of skill required to perform a procedure, along with a historical record of the amounts charged for that procedure. Although the consensus system covers a broader base of circumstances, it tends to be more slanted toward the creator of the system.

Fee-based Relative Value Systems

The fee-based RVS is a collection of databased on average fees charged for each procedure and sorted from highest to lowest. Then relative values are given according to a ratio of highest to lowest fee. Although a fee-based system appears to be more realistic than the consensus-based system, it is often hard to determine the accuracy of the database that was used, since it often is derived from data that were wrong in the first place because of computer conversions and the like.

Resource-Based Relative Value Systems

The third type of RVS is the resource-based relative value system (RBRVS), which takes into consideration the resources needed to provide a service or procedure. Its only current use is for Medicare reimbursement. Although the RBRVS takes into account the amount of physician work required, the actual expense of providing the service, the geographic area and malpractice expenses, it has led to numerous discrepancies and appears to have actually increased the volume of services rendered.

Regardless of the inadequacies that may be found in relative value systems, they provide a practice with a number of assets, the most important of which is a logical and objective method by which to calculate fees and defend those fees to the public and the payer. These systems also provide the ability to determine the procedures or services that are being rendered at a loss and generate a database that can be used to negotiate contractual care contracts.

Contract-Based Reimbursement

The methodology used by most HMOs, PPOs, and IPAs is the contract-based reimbursement schedule. It can be based on a percentage of the physician's usual charge, a preestablished fixed amount for a specific procedure or service, or a sliding scale based on the volume of patients. A host of possibilities exist for capitative care. There are almost as many varieties of contract-based reimbursement methods as there are organizations using them, and just when you think you've seen every possible variation, something new will turn up.

Percentage Reimbursement

The concept of paying a percentage of the physician's charge initially started with the onset of HMOs, which offered to supply volume in return for a discount. From the beginning, many of those contractual discounts were relatively small, amounting to only 5 or 10 percent. As HMOs grew in terms of the number of individuals covered, their cash needs became greater and those percentage discounts grew quite rapidly. In the majority of situations, there was nothing scientific about the size of the discount. More often than not, it simply a matter of supply and demand.

Fixed Fee Reimbursement

A need for fixed fee reimbursement for certain procedures grew out of the fact that in virtually every medical specialty there were always procedures performed for which the differential between the lowest fee and the highest fee was significant. For purposes of statistical budgeting, it became much easier to negotiate a fixed price for those procedures so that they might be performed for a level of reimbursement that was higher than expected or lower than expected, creating an overall average of satisfactory reimbursement.

Sliding Scale Reimbursement

The method of reimbursement known as sliding scales has evolved over many years. The most common form of sliding scale reimbursement is one in which a contract states that a certain defined amount will be paid for a given number of procedures. If a practitioner exceed that number, an additional discount will be taken for the procedures above that number or some form of rebate will be paid to a practitioner for going beyond that number.

Capitative Care

In recent years the concept of capitative care has been receiving greater acceptance in many areas. It is described by many as a pure "shared risk" concept, with the majority of risk falling to the practitioner. A deal is struck between an entity, an insurer, and a practitioner that offers a fixed number of individuals with a group plan and offers a fixed amount of money per month for each of those lives. In turn, a healthcare provider must provide those patients with any needed services within the provider's specialty. Because the insurer is simply taking up the monthly premiums and budgeting that amount, the majority of the risk lies with the practitioner. Most practitioners do not have access to the statistical demographics of a group of patients or know how many of them may need his or her services in a given month. There are other twists and turns to this concept, such as carve-outs, in which certain procedures are identified and an additional dollar amount is given to the practitioner if that procedure is necessary.

Negotiating Contractual Relationships

Whatever form contract-based reimbursement takes, it all comes back to the importance of managing one's A/R. In the following pages we will take a brief look at some of the things a practitioner can and should do when negotiating and overseeing contractual relationships. Although there are numerous books on negotiating a healthcare contract, here are several rules that I believe are important.

Rule 1. Have Ability To Monitor

In coming up with contract provisions, make sure you have the resources and abilities to monitor those provisions. For example, in the early days of discounted fees it was common practice to suggest to a practitioner that if he or she gave a discount, he or she should have the right to eliminate the discount if a procedure wasn't paid within a given time frame. After all, the enticement was that in return for treating those individuals at a discount, payment would be made much faster. As simple as that seems, the majority of practices do not have provisions to monitor that form of contractual relationship, let alone take corrective action. Also, many discount systems no longer use a simple percentage but a complex method to calculate the fee. Again, most practitioners don't have the capacity to keep a log of what the correct payment should be. Therefore, it is possible that the payer will pay less than what was in the original agreement simply because the practitioner didn't have the tools to monitor it. Finally, one must be aware of the cost that will be incurred for submitting additional claims if the entity does not keep its end of the bargain and provide timely reimbursements. This of course adds to staff time and to the probable cost of updating your billing system to monitor your contractual relationship.

Rule 2. Prepare for Change

Make sure you understand that the population you have agreed to treat can change. For example, you are approached by a local entity and enter into a contract. Thirty days later that firm is sold to a national entity, and rather than dealing with someone in your locale about the terms of your contract, you find yourself calling to the other side of the country to resolve problems. In a variation on this scenario, you initially joined this local entity because many of your patients were insured by it and it had a central processing center. All of a sudden it joins a much larger system with untold IPAs under its umbrella and claims to have little responsibility for enforcing the terms of your contract with the IPA.

Rule 3. Designate a Liaison

With these contractual relationships it is important to have someone in your practice who will be the liaison for those contracts. By the same token, during negotiations there is nothing wrong with asking the payer for a liaison who is reachable and in a position to correct those items that are not going appropriately.

Rule 4. Right of Termination

There can be numerous pitfalls in contracts for managed care. Although there may be a lot of pressure on your practice to sign up, there are some basic provisions that will be essential to your survival, especially the right of termination for failure to perform by the payer.

Overseeing Contractual Relationships

Regardless of what comes out of that negotiation, you need to be conscious of two things: receiving reimbursements that are lower than what you contracted for and the inability for review or recourse in the case of slow-paying contractual relationships.

Getting Less Than What Was Agreed Upon

The first rule in negotiating a contract is that a practice should have the ability to monitor reimbursements to make sure they are within the terms of the contract. Ideally, it is best to have software that can track managed care reimbursement daily, which very few practices have. If a practice is able to check these reimbursements, it may find the reimbursements received are lower than what the contractual agreement called for. If this is so, liaison to talk to about these discrepancies and then review and correct them.

Slow Reimbursement

The second arena that deserves attention is controlling slow reimbursement. Normally one enters into a contract with the assumption that because of greater cash turnaround, a larger discount can be taken by the payer for managed care. In most areas of the country that has proved to be mistaken. Again, it is imperative to have software to document payments as they relate to the age of an account. One should give extra attention to the contract in regard to this matter. Many contracts have clauses allowing the payer to put in any claim for a special review. Obviously, that could be all the claims. Therefore, consideration should be given to putting in a clause stating that 90 percent of all claims will be paid within 90 days.

Reimbursement Without Recourse

It is important that the contract not exclude you from pursuing other methods for collecting when the payer is not paying, such as the ability to notify a patient or the state insurance commissioner. In some cases it is worthwhile to contact the employer. This concept, however, needs special consideration since at least three states—Illinois, Maryland, and Florida—forbid a practitioner, the practitioner's billing company, or a collection agency from pursuing the debt in any way.

Summary

There is no question that managed care and capitation will become more prevalent. For a practice to exist in such an environment, a number of precautions must be taken. First, a practitioner has to know a lot more about his or her practice and the actual cost factors for each procedure and service rendered. More important, it is necessary to have some way to document those figures. When it comes time to negotiate for managed care or capitation, the physician with the most extensive knowledge of his or her practice will be in the best position. It is also important that a physician monitor managed care contracts, have a designated liaison to oversee them, be prepared for changes, and reserve the right to terminate a contract that has been unsuccessful.

Even though a practitioner may not have entered into a contractual relationship with an insurance entity, the concept of U&C is thrust upon the practitioner daily and he or she must be prepared to deal with the problems it can cause. Whether it is a matter of low reimbursement, slow pay, or reimbursement without recourse, a practitioner must be prepared to refuse to accept a provision yet still maintain good overall public relations.

A medical practice has to become proactive not just for the usual and customary problems but for all aspects that put the payer between the practitioner and the patient.

CHAPTER 10

SELECTING AND USING A THIRD PARTY COLLECTION AGENCY

The use of a third party agency for the collection of delinquent accounts is inevitable in most practices. However, since a collection agency is an extension of a practice, the utmost care must be taken to choose one that reflects the attitudes and philosophies of a practice to people who have ongoing financial obligations to that practice. Therefore, with regard to public relations, it is important that an agency have the ability to counsel patients as well as collect money. This ability is long remembered by financially over-burdened patient. It may not be reflected in the check the agency delivers each month, but in the long run it does pay. Patients who are indebted may be confused and belligerent, but few are dishonest. That is why an agency with a plan to help these people can be more important to a practice than is an agency that will do anything to collect. Once one accepts the fact that using a collection agency is a necessary part of effective A/R management, the process of selecting and working with an agency becomes elementary.

The 70-30 Rule

Unfortunately, many business managers exert all their efforts to ensure that the office collects every single account, and in the process they lose sight of the 70-30 rule (Figure 10-1). This rule states that 70 percent of patients voluntarily pay their bills or at least help make sure that payment is secured from a third party payer. Among the remaining patients, two-thirds will pay if they are persistently contacted by the entity to which they are indebted. The final 10 percent will not pay regardless of what steps are taken. Unfortunately, many practices give too much effort and time to the 10 percent that is uncollectible and fail to give full attention to the 90 percent that is collectible. Sometimes,

Figure 10-1: 70-30 Rule

70% of patients voluntarily pay their bills
20% of patients will pay if persistently contacted
10% of patients will not pay no matter what

---

this becomes a personal crusade to collect every dollar, but if the aged accounts are referred to a professional debt collector (a collection agency), it becomes a business transaction instead of an emotional experience. The collector does not become personally involved, will not express anger that may damage public relations, and remembers the 70-30 rule.

The Collection Agency As An Extension Of The Practice

As stated in the opening paragraph of this chapter, a healthcare provider is selecting an extension of itself in choosing a collection agency. It must seek out an agency that reflects its own philosophy. However, healthcare providers should remember that collection agencies are governed by the Federal Fair Debt Collection Practices Act (see Chapter 7), which prohibits the use of abusive tactics by debt collectors. A practice should obtain reasonable assurance that the agency selected adheres to those provisions and to any state laws that are applicable.

In addition, the collection agency should have the same level of professionalism as the healthcare provider. In other words, the practice should seek out agencies that operate in an ethical manner not merely because of federal regulations, but because of an inherent belief in their own industry. Not only does a professional collector want to recover dollars for a practice, with a contingency fee as the incentive, he or she is there to give help and direction to patients who may be overburdened by financial worries. A truly professional collector knows how to help debtors settle their financial troubles.

When a collection agency is selected, both the practice and the agency must recognize that there has to be two-way communication and support for the relationship to be mutually satisfactory. When delinquent accounts are turned over to the collection agency, a practice has released them and given the agency full responsibility for them. If a patient contacts a practitioner a week after the account was placed with an agency, pleading to make a "deal," the practitioner must explain that an effort was made to resolve the outstanding balance with the patient many times before and now it is in the hands of the collection agency. The collection agency must reciprocate this trust and responsibility by providing confirmation of placements and timely month-end reports to the practice.

Types of Agencies

Before beginning the process of selecting a professional debt collector, you must understand that there are different types of agencies. Although their goals may be identical, the collection methods they use and the way they are reimbursed are different. The three types of agencies are prepaid agencies, law firms, and full-service collection agencies.

Prepaid Agencies

In this arrangement, a practice purchases coupons from an agency which it will later use to list delinquent accounts. Prepaid agencies use several variations of the coupon program. Agencies of this type tend to have a national headquarters with many satellite offices and often are strictly letter-writing services, although some do telephone contact as well.

A practice should ask for clarification about the services a prepaid agency performs. In some cases prepaid agencies stipulate in the contract that unless the creditor can furnish a current address for the debtor, the agency will hold the account in abeyance. This means that the agency does not do skip tracing. Since studies have shown that 20 percent of the populace relocates each year, effective collection work is dependent on skip tracing. Since the average practice does not have the time or tools to do this, it is important that the agency supply this service.

Usually, the more coupons a practice purchases, the lower the cost of the individual coupon. The danger lies in the temptation to purchase more coupons than necessary. If the practice becomes dissatisfied with the agency's work, there may be no way to redeem the unused coupons. A practitioner should also be aware that some prepaid agencies use endorsements from local medical societies which to create the impression that this service is offered by the medical society rather than by an independent contractor. It is vital to clarify the nature of such implied relationships.

Law Firms

The introduction of the federal Fair Debt Collection Practices Act, which was aimed at collection agencies but did not apply to attorneys, caused a proliferation of agencies to form which were staffed by a single attorney, with several employees who were not attorneys actually doing the collection work. In the summer of 1986 attorneys were brought under the control of the FDCPA; this means that they are no longer exempt and have no more power than does a regular collection agency.

Law firms normally charge a contingency fee that is based on the success of the collection effort. If the case goes to litigation, court costs are usually collected in advance; this means that the practitioner is making an investment in the hopes that the attorney will be successful. If the healthcare provider chooses a law firm to collect its delinquent accounts, it should give serious consideration to finding one with which it can readily communicate and one that is familiar with the culture and customs of the area.

Full-Service Collection Agencies

The professional full-service debt collection agency traditionally solicits business on a contingency basis and performs all facets of the collection effort, including precollection packages, skip tracing, and litigation. It may be locally based or part of a national chain. Its contingency fees often are assessed on a sliding scale that is based on the age of the account and the dollar amount and volume of the business. In many cases extra fees may be charged for additional efforts required in the collection process, such as forwarding the account to an agency in another area.

Selecting A Collection Agency

The requirements for selecting a reputable prepaid agency, law firm, or full-service collection agency are relatively simple. However, all of the following steps, not just those which come easily, should be taken.

Create a List of Available Agencies

There are several ways to find available agencies. First and foremost is word of mouth. Ask other healthcare practitioners in the area about their experiences with collection agencies. Agencies can also be found in the classified section of local phone books. A phone call to a trade associations for referrals is another possibility.

Obtain Information About the Agencies on Your List

An easy way to learn about an agency is to send its manager a simple questionnaire. The same questionnaire can be sent to several agencies so that they all can respond on an equal basis. The questionnaire should be structured to include pertinent questions such as "How long have you been in business?" "What is the smallest size account you will accept for placement?" "How long do you normally work an account?" and "At what point do you make the first telephone call?"

It is important to ask whether the agency is affiliated or is a member of a professional trade associations. The three best known trade associations in the collection industry are Medical-Dental-Hospital Bureaus of America (MDHBA), the American Collectors Association (ACA), and the Associated Credit Bureaus of America (ACBA), Collection Division. Membership in one or all of these trade associations will not guarantee a perfect agency, but it will indicate that the agency adheres to a code of ethics and probably is actively involved in continuing education about changes in the collection industry as they pertain to the healthcare field.

If at all possible it would be beneficial to use a collection agency that has been certified through an association's program. For example, Medical-Dental-Hospital Business Associates has an education program that will license a business as a "Certified Health Care Collection Agency." From personal experience working for a company that has received its certification I can tell you the process takes a lot of work. At the same time, an agency with the certification will be on the cutting edge of health care collection and will be better equipped to meet the needs of the health care provider.

Whatever questions are included on the questionnaire, an assessment is made of each potential agency on the basis of the same information. Once the field of candidates has been narrowed, you should solicit requests for proposals from those who are on your "preferred list."

Check with the State to Confirm Licensing

Many states have licensing requirements for collection agencies, and in most of them, licensing is handled by the department of registration and education. Appendix B contains a list of states that have licensing requirements and their licensing administrators and a list of the licensing administrators for all the Canadian provinces. Check with the appropriate department to verify that the agency is licensed and whether any formal complaints have been filed against it.

Make an Appointment to Visit the Agency's Office

It is essential for a practitioner to meet the principals of any agency that may represent the practice. An on-site visit can tell a great deal about an agency. If possible, try to observe the agency's total operation and don't hesitate to ask to observe a collector at work. During the visit, discuss what the agency will and will not do during the process of collection. For example, find out how it accepts transfer of account information. Does a listing sheet have to be completed for each account, or is it possible to utilize tape-to-tape or diskette-to-diskette transfer? Some agencies send someone from the staff to a physician's office to photostat account information.

Collection agencies may want a signed contract or agreement, although this is not always necessary. If a written contract is requested, it should include provision for withdrawals of accounts, such as the circumstances under which they are allowed and the fee or penalty that may be imposed. In the interview process, the collection agency will want to see representative examples of a practice's billing statements. It will probably ask at what point in the collection process a delinquent account is normally listed with an agency. If a contract is signed, it must be reasonable for both parties.

Evaluate the Rates Charged by Each Agency on Your List

If an on-site visit was made to each collection agency, along with a background check of the licensing, the list of potential candidates should be shorter. The final step is to evaluate the rates the candidates charge. The contingency percentage—the amount a collection agency charges for the successful collection of an account—is one way to compare agencies. However, in effective A/R management, the primary concern is the yield gained: the net amount of money that comes back to a practice from accounts that have been placed with a professional debt collector.

For example, if two seemingly identical agencies were offering full collection services, one at a contingency rate of 40 percent and the other at a rate of 30 percent, it would be natural to opt for the one with the 30 percent rate. However, if the firm with the higher contingency rate had a recovery rate of 40 percent and the agency with the lower contingency rate had a recovery rate of 20 percent, about two-thirds of a practice's yield would be lost by using the agency with the lower recovery rate. Figure 10-2 shows what would happen if both agencies received $10,000 worth of placements from the same practitioner.

Developing A Request For Proposal

The most objective and effective way of choosing a professional collection agency is to develop a request for proposal and distribute it to several agencies which have met your other criteria. A request for proposal (RFP) is a formal document that may be several pages long and that asks for specific information about the agency and how it operates. It invites an agency to submit a detailed application describing the services it provides and explain how it would handle the healthcare provider's collection business. Each agency in contention for the business receives the same RFP, which lists information about the

Figure 10-2: Comparing Collection Agencies by Yield

	Agency A	Agency B
$10,000 worth of placements with a contingency rate of	30%	40%
Recovery percentage	20%	35%
Total recovered	$2,000	$3,500
Minus commission	$600	$1,400
Net back	$1,400	$2,100

healthcare provider and the type of practice and gives an indication of the approximate volume of delinquent accounts that will be placed monthly. It also describes the collection work that is open for bidding. The RFP is sent to firms that you have determined are qualified. Appendix C shows a sample RFP. Here are some essential elements that should be included in an RFP:

1. *Purpose of the Request*: a short statement describing the project and the level of authorization for the request.

2. *Description of the organization making the request*: general information about the healthcare provider, including a practice profile, annual charges and receipts, an organizational chart, long-range plans, and operating characteristics such as the type of data processing equipment used.

3. *Description of the Service Needed*: a detailed summary of what kind of services are to be expected, along with an outline of the practice's billing cycle, how delinquent accounts are handled, and when they are turned over for collection. There also should be an estimated starting date for the work to begin.

4. *Information about the Collection Agency*: a description of the agency and how it operates. Here is a list of criteria that should be included in this portion of the RFP:

   - What the collection agency will do with an account

   - A brief background of the company

   - Qualifications of the firm

   - Client references

   - Number of employees and their qualifications

   - Estimated fees and payment terms expected

5. *Information regarding Submittal of the Proposal*: the date when the proposal is due, the number of copies desired, and where the proposal is to be sent.

Evaluating A Request For Proposal

Once the RFPs have been sent out and proposals have been returned by the collection agencies, the process of reviewing the proposals begins. To help evaluate a proposal in a uniform fashion, the American Collectors Association, through its Healthcare Services Program, has developed a Request for Proposal Rating Scale (Figure 10-3). This system of rating RFPs allows for evaluation in six areas, with a certain number of points allotted to each area.

Figure 10-3: Request for Proposal Rating Scale

REQUEST FOR PROPOSAL
RATING SCALE

	Possible	Score
ORGANIZATION OF AGENCY - 17 POINTS		
1. Length of time in business	5	_____
2. Financial stability	5	_____
3. Experience servicing same type of business	2	_____
4. Continuing education of agency employees	2	_____
5. Organization (size and qualifications of staff)	1	_____
6. Size of agency	1	_____
7. Geographic area serviced	1	_____
SERVICES PROVIDED - 32 POINTS		
1. Automation, 12 points		
a. Trust accounting	2	_____
b. Current technology	5	_____
c. On-line services	5	_____
2. Management reports, 10 points		
a. Debtor status	5	_____
b. Statistical analyses	5	_____
3. Training of client's employees	3	_____
4. Precollect system	2	_____
5. Volume of accounts handled yearly	2	_____
6. Collection procedure for each account	2	_____
7. Service representative	1	_____
RATES - 20 POINTS		
1. Contingent fee	10	_____
2. Step rate based on type/volume/age	10	_____
RECOVERY PERCENTAGE - 14 POINTS		
Recovery percentage	14	_____
OTHER - 17 POINTS		
1. Insurance of adequate amounts, 7 points		
a. Professional liability	3	_____
b. Employee fidelity	2	_____
c. General liability	2	_____
2. References	2	_____
3. Membership in trade and professional associations	2	_____
4. Ability to protect client from liability	2	_____
5. Completeness of proposal	4	_____
TOTAL POINTS	**100**	_____

Adapted from Healthcare Client Services program of the American Collectors Association

The six areas for judging proposals are: agency organization, services, rates, recovery percentage, other insurance coverage and references, and discretionary. For example, the recovery percentage of a collection agency can earn up to 14 points, the contingency fee up to 10 points, and the length of time in business up to 5 points, while the size of the agency is worth only 1 point. After all the proposals have been scored, an impartial judgement can be made of which collection agency is the best. Obviously, a collection agency that scores 90 points is going to look better than a collection agency that only scores 60 points, even though the contingency rate of the lower scoring agency is far lower than that of the higher scoring agency.

What To Expect From A Collection Agency

Once a collection agency has been selected, a number of things should be expected from that agency. Remember that a collection agency is an agent representing a practice. As we stated previously, it is an extension of a practice and should reflect the ethics and standards of that practice. With that in mind, one should expect a collection agency to do the following:

1. *Scrupulously observe all federal and state laws in collecting the account.* These laws were designed to protect the consumer. If it abides by them, a collection agency has less exposure to lawsuits, which can affect the reputation of a practice.

2. *Start work immediately on the accounts.* Within 7 days of placement, the first contact should have been made with a debtor and the collection process should have been launched.

3. *Remit all the proceeds from the collections made, minus the appropriate fee, once a month.*

4. *Provide a detailed list of the debtors from whom money has been collected, the dates of collection, the amounts collected, and the balance still due.*

5. *Provide regular progress or debtor status reports.*

6. *Promptly and fairly handle disputed accounts to determine whether the dispute has any validity.*

7. *Not start legal action against a debtor unless the law permits and the practice gives written authorization to do so.*

8. *Review the practice's A/R management system.*

9. *Help train the practice's staff in techniques for dealing with credit and collection problems.*

What A Collection Agency Expects In Return

Once a collection agency has been chosen, it should be treated as a full partner, with trust, loyalty, and support. It should feel it has the opportunity to serve a practice and that the practice will not go to another firm unless the agency deviates from ethical standards. A good agency's peak of recovery will come later. A practice should trust an agency to work in the best interests of the practice and always keep the lines of communication open.

An agency wants and expects to hear from a practice that has become dissatisfied. If an agency is not working to the full satisfaction of a practice, it wants to know. As a partner, the agency will act quickly to clear up misunderstandings and problems. In addition to these basic guidelines, an agency also expects a practice to do the following things.

Provide Complete Information

To ensure that a collector will do the best job, as much information as possible about the account must be provided. This information includes

- All pertinent information from the patient information for.

- The correct amount owed, including any payments, interest, or late charges that have been added

- On a skip case, any skip tracing work that has been done

- On a disputed account, all the information about the complaint

- Whether the account had previously been placed with another collection agency and returned uncollected

In regards to bankruptcy cases, it is imperative that the collection agency be notified immediately, because continuing collection efforts in a bankruptcy case is a violation of federal bankruptcy laws.

Give the Collection Agency Full Responsibility

Once an account has been assigned to an agency for collection, it is vital that the agency be given full responsibility for handling it. If a debtor contacts a practice after receiving notification that the account is in the hands of a collection agency, it is imperative that the practice refer that person to the agency. Accept no compromise arrangements and do not agree to discontinue collection efforts. Remind the patient that a great effort has been made to work things out and that it is now necessary to work directly with the collection agency to resolve the account.

Promptly Notify Your Collector If Direct Payment is Received

Often debtors mail payments directly to the practice, not to the collection agency. When this occurs, the collection agency should be notified right away or the payment should be mailed to the collection agency immediately to ensure that the debtor is credited with the payment and that its collection efforts are modified accordingly.

Pay The Collection Agency Promptly

Although in most cases a collection agency is paid by deducting its commissions from the amount it collects and sending the net amount to the practice, occasionally a practice may owe the agency money, usually because of a large volume of direct payments. Sometimes a practice will arrange for a collection agency to send it the gross proceeds and then issue a check to the agency for its commissions. The partnership is built on trust, and it is only fair that an agency to be paid in a timely manner.

Evaluating And Monitoring A Collection Agency's Performance

It is important that a healthcare provider have a way to track a collection agency's effectiveness. This audit process can be done by keeping a log book which shows the number of accounts placed with an agency and their dollar amount on a month-to-month basis. In this log the practice should keep track of the agency's month-end results by tracking the gross collections. In a short time, an agency's collection percentage, or net collection, can be calculated by dividing the gross collections by gross placements for a particular period. Many agencies will subtract all accounts that are returned for any reason, and this increases the percentage.

For example, if practice A placed $40,000 worth of placements with agency B during the first 6 months of a given year and agency B collected $9,200, after returning $2,500 during those 6 months, the agency would have a collection percentage of 24.5 percent, which would be considered average. In the healthcare field, the average collection rate achieved by collection agencies is approximately 24 percent. Obviously, if the collection percentage of an agency is below that, an explanation would be expected from the collection agency's management. It may be discovered that the demographic information given to the agency was incomplete or incorrect. If the collection percentage of an agency is high, such as 40 percent, one needs to look at the internal operations of the practice because this is a sign that accounts are being turned over to an agency too rapidly.

Another tactic is to call an agency's manager and ask to review a few accounts at the collection agency's offices. Selecting accounts at random and reviewing the action that has been taken not only can give a practitioner a better view of the work that has been done on an account but also gives the practitioner a chance to supply additional information about the account that may assist the agency in its recovery efforts. In addition, the manager of the agency can later convey to the collectors what has taken place during the review. In the physician's office as well as in the collection agency, it is best if there are predefined terms for what will be used as a measurement for judging success.

Collection Key Terms

Following are some terms used by professional debt collectors which may differ from standard definitions.

Assets

When used by a collection agency, one of the ingredients necessary for litigation. One must find assets of a debtor to make a case for litigation. If the debtor has no known assets, it is fruitless to file suit.

Contingency

The percentage fee charged by the collection agency for the money actually collected.

Demographics

Information obtained about a debtor, including name, address, employer, and phone numbers. The better the demographics, the better the chances for recovery.

Derogatory Information

Normally this is the information that a collection agency reports to a credit bureau in regards to the delinquency of a debtor. Once the debt is paid, the derogatory information must be reversed or removed from the credit report of the debtor.

Early Out

A product sold by some collection agencies primarily to hospitals and large clinics by which after a predetermined number of days (normally 90), the account automatically moves to a collection agency for a specified follow-up procedure, such as a letter or phone call. This is a modification of a precollection program.

Net Back

The amount of money actually returned to the credit granter or the amount collected minus the contingency fee. More often than not it is not so much the fee charged but the actual yield that is of primary importance.

Paid Direct

A payment made directly to a client as opposed to one made to an agency.

PIF

Paid in full—the goal of all collection efforts.

Placement

Synonymous with the phrase "new business"—the accounts that are "placed" for collection.

Power dialer

An automatic phone dialer that dials numbers at a predetermined speed.

Precollection

A service available from many agencies that allows a credit granter to place accounts with an agency for one or two letters or for a letter and a phone call at a fixed fee. At the end of a set time period, if the account is not paid, it is handled as a regular collection account at normal contingency rates.

Predictive dialer

A new and sophisticated device that ties into an agency's computer, automatically dialing phone numbers at a predetermined rate. This can increase the individual collector's productivity.

Prepaid coupon

A coupon sold at a set price by some collection agencies. The credit granter redeems the coupon when an account is collected. There is normally a contingency fee over and above that cost.

Recovery

The amount of delinquent debt that is actually collected.

Retainer

In some situations, agencies charge a set monthly fee for a predetermined amount of work.

Skip

A debtor who moves without notifying creditors. Intentional skips move in order evade creditors.

Skip Tracing

The process of using various tools to locate skips and pursue collection efforts.

Summary

Almost every practice has to solicit the help of a professional debt collector at some time. It has been shown that 70 percent of Americans voluntarily pay their medical bills. Of the remaining 30 percent, one-third have no intention of paying. However, the remaining twenty percent will pay if they are coaxed correctly. This is where a professional debt collector becomes valuable. The collection of delinquent accounts is a business transaction for the collection agency, not an emotional experience, as be the case in a practice.

However, since a collection agency is an extension of a practice, the utmost care must be taken to choose one that reflects the attitudes and philosophies of the practice. There are three types of collection agencies: prepaid agencies, law firms, and full-service collection agencies. Most common are full-service collection agencies, which perform all aspects of collection work and charge a contingency fee only if they are successful in their collection efforts.

There are several steps to take in selecting a collection agency. First, get a list of available agencies either by asking colleagues or contacting a trade association for collection agencies. Second, make an appointment and physically visit the collection agencies that are in competition for your business. Third, develop a request for proposal (RFP), which is a lengthy list of questions and comments about a collection agency and its fees and an explanation of the services desired. When the proposals are received, evaluate them by using an RFP rating scale.

Once a collection agency has been chosen, there are certain things a practice can expect from that agency, such as abiding by federal and state laws, working accounts immediately, remitting collections monthly, and providing detailed reports of placements, remittances, and balances remaining. In return, a collection agency can expect a practice to treat it as a full partner. A collection agency has the right to be informed if a practice is dissatisfied for any reason. In addition, a collection agency needs to have all pertinent information about the account, including any disputes or complaints by patients. Once an account is assigned to a collection agency, the agency must retain full control over the account, without interference from the practice. A practice should evaluate and monitor the effectiveness of a collection agency from time to time by tracking its net collection percentage.

By investing a small amount of time and following the recommendations outlined here, a healthcare provider can be assured of a successful long-term relationship with a professional debt collection agency.

CHAPTER 11

HIPAA COMPLIANCE AND ACCOUNTS RECEIVABLE

HIPAA is the acronym for the Health Insurance Portability and Accountability Act, which was passed by Congress in 1996 and is due to be fully implemented by 2003. Its implementation will affect the way health care providers and their business associates, which includes medical billing and accounts receivable management companies, operate.

Background

HIPAA has two main provisions. The first is portability of health care insurance (transferring health insurance from one employer to another). This became an important political issue in the 1990s when health care costs continued to rise, and increasing numbers of Americans found themselves uninsured. Title I of HIPAA protects health insurance coverage for workers and their families when they change or lose jobs, or when they have pre-existing conditions. It prohibits discrimination by health insurance carriers based on the health status of the insured.

The second major provision is Administrative Simplification (HIPAA Title II). It is this provision that will most affect your practice. This provision encourages health plans, health care clearinghouses, and health care providers to conduct financial and administrative transactions electronically. Title II of HIPAA authorized the Department of Health and Human Services (HHS) to establish national uniform standards to facilitate the electronic transmission of data in health care transactions. This includes code sets to describe the data and national identification numbers for providers, employers, and health plans. This was done to improve the effectiveness and efficiency of the nation's health care system.

An important component of Administrative Simplification is patient privacy (the Privacy Rule). With the increase in electronic transmission of health care data and the rapid growth of health care systems technology came the concern for protecting the confidentiality of an individual's health information. The underlying concept of patient privacy legislation is that no patient information should be released to any entity without the express written consent of the patient, and only then the information should be released to an entity that abides by the privacy rules. The privacy protections are intended to assure consumers that their health information, including genetic information, will be properly protected.

Under the Privacy Rule, health plans, health care clearinghouses, and certain health care providers must guard against misuse of individuals' identifiable health information, and limit sharing of such information. Since medical billing companies must use individually identifiable health information, they must be responsible for helping maintain confidentiality. Health care providers and their business associates must comply with the Act. This may create additional costs of doing business and may potentially cause unintended effects on health care delivery and access for individuals.

Patient Privacy

Historically, patient health care information has been released without the patient's authorization or knowledge. In the mid-1990s, patient privacy advocates used the media to create awareness of this issue. Most of the time the release of patient information was merely a by-product of conducting business and did no harm. However, sometimes information was inappropriately disclosed. As a result, all health care professionals and their business associates were portrayed by the media as destroying a patients' right to privacy. With the advent of electronic billing, keeping patient information private became an increasingly difficult dilemma.

Early versions of HIPAA tried to address the patient privacy issue, but the legislation was uninformed in health care practices and this legislation did not make it out of the Senate review committees. The process for HIPAA has been a lengthy one, and refinements and changes in the legislation are continually being made. There is an ongoing attempt to balance the business needs of health care providers with the necessity of protecting patient information.

Many health care-related trade associations are actively seeking changes in HIPAA legislation. With all the changes that HIPAA proposes for electronic transmission of information and patient privacy, many health care providers and their business associates feel that in trying to comply, their businesses would be undermined financially. They argue that HIPAA will cause more work, raise fees, and have a negative impact on the availability of services. For collection agencies, medical billing businesses, and practices alike, updating software, training employees, and signing nondisclosure agreements with vendors and clients could be very expensive. As a result, HIPAA will have a direct influence on the profitability of many of these businesses.

Key Terms

In order to comply with HIPAA one must understand the key terms of which there are many. One version of the HIPAA glossary was 24 pages long and averaged 20 definitions a page. These few definitions listed here cover the most important concepts.

Covered Entity

A health care organization, a health care clearinghouse, or a health care provider who transmits patient health information electronically is considered a "covered entity" and must comply with this Act. For the time being, "patient health information" is considered any patient information. As such, all health care providers who conduct business electronically can be considered covered entities. This also includes business associates or vendors contracted by health care providers, those who render a service to covered entities but are not directly employed by the provider, HMOs, health insurance plans, health care clearinghouses, Medicare, and Medicaid.

Health Information

Oral or recorded patient information that is in any medium.

Protected Health Information (PHI)

Information sent electronically as defined in part 45 CFR 162.103 of HIPAA. This would include any and all health care information regarding a patient.

Individually Identifiable Health Information (IIHI)

This is a subset of an individual patient's health information. It includes patient demographic information and any personal information created or received by a provider or it's business associate that can identify an individual patient.

Business Associate (BA)

A person or organization that performs a function or activity on behalf of a covered entity, but is not part of the covered entity's workforce. A business associate is any entity that is not an employee of the covered entity, but performs a function that uses patient information. A business associate can also be a covered entity in its own right. The following are some types of business associates:

 Billing Services

 Utilization review services

 Coding services

 Legal services

 Practice management services

 Transcription services

 Business Associate Agreements

This requirement says that if a covered entity creates personal health information for a patient and gives it to another party, there must be an agreement between the two parties about how that information will be used. More importantly is how the information will be protected and used for only the purpose that it was revealed. This written contract or agreement must comply with 45 CFR 164.504[e] which requires a business associate to create and implement a compliance program.

It is the responsibility of the party creating the data to ensure that its vendors are upholding the business associate agreements. This responsibility also pertains to the termination of an agreement with a business partner. Termination procedures that are in compliance with HIPAA will need to be defined in the compliance plan and written into the agreements.

Chain of Trust Agreement

Type of contract that extends the responsibility to protect health care data across a series of sub-contractual relationships. Using the last definition to give one the depth that these rules go, many believe it will be necessary to have Business Associate Agreements with anyone that would have access to space where medical information was kept in an accessible location. For example, a medical file left open on a desk after-hours may result in a need to have an agreement with the cleaning service.

Electronic Transactions and Electronic Signatures

This establishes standard data content, codes, and formats for submitting electronic claims. Your software will need to be able to support the ANSI X12 format. If you use a clearinghouse or third party medical biller, a Business Associate Agreement will need to be in place. Although compliance with the standards was initially due October 16, 2002 an extension can be obtained until October 16, 2003. To receive this extension the covered entity needs to submit a plan as to how it will achieve compliance by the new deadline. You can find a sample compliance plan and get an extension form online from Centers for Medicare and Medicaid Services (CMS) at http://www.cms.hhs.gov/hipaa/hipaa2/ascaform.asp.

Privacy Standards

This is by far the most complex element of HIPAA; it addresses the individual's rights regarding "identifiable health information." Key to this will be the form given to the patient before treatment, which explains those rights and tells them who will have access to the information and how it is protected. Compliance to this element is due April 14, 2003.

Patient Release Form

HIPAA requires providers to give patients a clear and written explanation of how their personal information will be used and maintained, and to whom it will be disclosed. The form must not be attached to other documents and must explain the patient's rights.

Security standards

Although the final security standards have not been released, they will define how electronic data is transmitted and how improper access should be monitored and stopped. Also defined within this element is the availability of health information that is not individually identifiable. It will dictate to what degree you are responsible to prevent a third party from obtaining information that they are not entitled to use.

Implementation

Practices, hospitals, and their business associates will need a HIPAA compliance plan in order to comply with the federal rules. The legislation does not describe how this should be done, but safeguarding data, office policies, and employee training are the critical key points. The idea is that everyone will be compliant by 2004, but many practices will still have difficulty in complying by the deadlines. Each element has had different deadlines and each of those has changed. April 2003 now appears to be final for the largest of the elements, patient privacy.

How a practice takes the first step towards implementation will depend greatly on its size and existing office structure. What procedures your office already has in place will be an indication of how much your office will need to be restructured. For example, if your office already shreds documents rather than putting them in a wastebasket, you will be one step closer to implementation than a practice that does not shred its documents.

Resources

Most answers regarding HIPAA implementation questions can be found at the Department of Health and Human Services (HHS) website (http://www.dhhs.gov/). Also on the HHS website are fact sheets that explain different aspects of HIPAA and Patient Privacy. A list is located at http://www.hhs.gov/news/facts/. The Administration Simplification aspects of HIPAA are explained at http://aspe.os.dhhs.gov/admnsimp/. A very thorough question and answer FAQ sheet regarding Administration Simplification can be located at http://aspe.os.dhhs.gov/admnsimp/final/pvcguide1.htm. The Center for Medicare and Medicaid Services (CMS) website (http://www.cms.hhs.gov/hipaa/) has a comprehensive summary of HIPAA legislation in relation to Medicare and Medicaid.

Figure 11-1: Sample Patient's Rights Form

AUTHORIZATION FOR RELEASE OF INFORMATION

SECTION A: MUST BE COMPLETED FOR ALL AUTHORIZATIONS

I hereby authorize the use or disclosure of my health information as described below. I understand the information disclosed pursuant to this authorization may be subject to redisclosure by the recipient and no longer protected by federal privacy regulations.

Patient name: _____   ID Number: _____

Persons/organizations providing the information: Persons/organizations receiving the information:

_____   _____
_____   _____
_____   _____

Specific description of information (including date(s)): _____
_____
_____
_____

SECTION B: MUST BE COMPLETED ONLY IF THE HEALTHCARE PROVIDER HAS REQUESTED THE AUTHORIZATION

1.   The health plan or health care provider must complete the following:
    a.   What is the purpose of the use or disclosure? _____
           _____
    b.   Will the healthcare provider requesting the authorization receive financial or in-kind compensation in exchange for using or disclosing the health information described above?   Yes ___ No ___

2.   The patient or the patient's representative must read and initial the following statements:
    a.   I understand that my health care and the payment for my health care will not be affected if I do not sign this form.   Initials: _____
    b.   I understand that I may see and copy the information described on this form if I ask for it, and that I get a copy of this form after I sign it.   Initials: _____

SECTION C: MUST BE COMPLETED FOR ALL AUTHORIZATIONS

The patient or the patient's representative must read and initial the following statements:
1.   I understand that this authorization will expire on ___/___/___ (MM/DD/YY).   Initials: _____
2.   I understand that I may revoke this authorization at any time by notifying the healthcare provider in writing and that the revocation will be effective from the date it is received and will not apply retroactively.
           Initials: _____

_____   ___/___/___
Signature of patient or patient's representative   **Date**
(*THIS FORM MUST BE COMPLETED BEFORE SIGNING*)
Printed name of patient's representative: _____

Relationship to the patient: _____

YOU MAY REFUSE TO SIGN THIS AUTHORIZATION
You may not use this form to release information for treatment or payment except when the information to be released is psychotherapy notes or certain research information.

Many professional societies and trade associations have excellent assessment and requirement checklists available for very small fees. It would be worthwhile to contact one of these associations to see what they can provide.

Trade magazines and publishers have also put out specialty books to help with compliance. PMIC (http:\\www.pmiconline.com) has a very informative book on HIPAA implementation, *HIPAA Compliance Manual*. The American Medical Association has resources for its members as well (http:// www.ama-assn.org/).

There are also medical billing consultants available who can help with implementation, but their fees can be expensive. If time is more of a factor than money, then it may make more sense to hire a consultant instead of doing it yourself.

Staff Education

Staff education in the new regulations is essential. These are the individuals that will have to explain in an audit why your practice follows its procedures. Give your office and staff access to an internet newsgroup, subscribe to a professional or trade journal, or become a member of an association to receive timely, helpful, and relevant information. Both you and your staff should be up-to-date as much as possible with the latest news on HIPAA, its changing regulations, and how it affects job duties.

Compliance Officer

Your practice will need a HIPAA compliance officer. It will be the only way to ensure you're in compliance. This person can be an employee of the practice or a consultant. By designating a reasonably knowledgeable compliance officer early in the implementation process, you will have an informed person to help guide the process. This will save you many headaches later on.

Patient's Rights Form

After assigning a HIPAA compliance officer, a Patient's Rights form should be the next priority. Once the practice has it in place, it will help to make the other elements of the implementation plan fall into place. The Patient's Rights form should be short and written in plain language. It should inform the patient that his information may be disclosed for treatment and payment purposes, that the patient has the right to review the provider's privacy notice, and that he has the right to request restrictions and to revoke consent at anytime. There should be a space on the form for the patient to sign and date to show they know their rights and have given consent. A sample form is shown in Figure 11-1.

Associate Agreements

Business Associate Agreements will likely come from your vendor. Neither your collection agency nor your third party medical biller can do business with you if they do not have in place non-disclosure agreements. Since your vendor will likely need to sign contracts with many of its clients, it would be easier for you and less confusing for your vendor if you stick to their standard agreement. Contact your vendors to see what they have done about this element of implementation. Figure 11-2 outlines the elements that need to be present in any Business Associate Agreement. Make sure you thoroughly review any contract or agreement to make sure all the HIPAA requirements are present before signing it.

Safeguarding Patient Information

All patient data, electronic and paper, will need to be protected. Patient files will need to be in a secured area, either locking file cabinets or in a locked room. If your office is already using locking file cabinets you are well on your way to being compliant. Access by staff members should be limited to those who need to access the files on a regular basis. The fewer people who have keys to the cabinets the better. Computers that contain patient information should be accessible only by a password. Only those staff members who have a need should be able to access the information.

Figure 11-2: Key points for Business Associate Agreements

When reviewing a Business Agreement be sure that:

- Your office is clearly designated as the Covered Entity and your vendor is labeled as the Business Associate.

- Each company's responsibility in handling and disclosing of patient health information (PHI) is specified.

- The vendor details its safeguarding procedures for:

    —Receiving PHI from the Covered Entity

    —Processing PHI

    —Limiting disclosure of PHI to essential employees

    —Storing PHI

    —Destroying PHI

- The length of the agreement is specified.

- There is an Agreement Termination Plan that is acceptable to both parties. It should describe how the Business Associate will safeguard or dispose of patient information when the contract is terminated.

- In the case of a breach of contract by either party, there are steps described in the Agreement for actions to be taken.

Exchange of Electronic Data

Anyone in health care that uses electronic data will agree that standardizing the exchange of electronic data will improve efficiency and effectiveness. At the same time, better protection of the data will result from HIPAA legislation. However, if that means that no one can see the CPT code of a patient's encounter without a need, and your computer system software does not have firewalls for information protection, you may start to disagree. There are many systems in use that don't meet HIPAA requirements, and in many cases it's the big systems for hospitals, not just the solo practitioner that need to be updated. Since your office budget most likely has a sum allotted for computer upgrades, it would be prudent to increase that amount during the year you implement HIPAA for new computers or a new software system that will be able to meet HIPAA requirements for electronic data.

Getting Started

Start implementing HIPAA requirements while using resources already available to you.

- Designate an employee as the HIPAA compliance officer and allow time for that person to become well-informed on the subject.

- Contact your vendors for non-disclosure agreements.

- Keep abreast of new information and changes by joining a newsgroup.

- Talk to your peers to see how they are approaching HIPAA implementation.

- Update an old computer system to a HIPAA compliant system—something that probably needs to be done anyway.

- Create a Patient's Rights form for your office.

There is no way to comply with HIPAA completely without some cost, but by using resources that are already available and spending money on things for which you already budgeted, you should be able to comply for a nominal cost.

Enforcement and Penalties

No private actions can be taken according to HIPAA regulations, but there are civil penalties for violations. There is a $100 fine for each violation. Since there are so many sections to HIPAA and many that overlap, a single mistake could amount to multiple errors and be very costly. Federal criminal penalties for obtaining or improperly disclosing of information is a fine of $50,000 and one year in prison; if done under false pretenses the fine is $100,000 and five years in prison; and if done with the intent to benefit monetarily the fine is $250,000 and ten years in prison.

Summary

In 2001 enough material was published on HIPAA to fill a library, the number of HIPAA-related seminars offered would not fit into a year, and all this before the rules were even published. Most of the debate came from strict interpretations of the rules that sometimes seemed to be used as scare tactics. The discussion rarely focused on how physicians should *rationally* conduct their practices.

For instance, it was generally accepted that it would be a violation of the rules of patient privacy if there were any documentation connecting a patient's name to a physician's name. In that case, could a bulletin board in a pediatric practice wishing "happy birthday" to its patients be considered a violation? Another example would be a doctor's office accepting a check from a patient that had a memo written on it stating "office visit." When the check was deposited into the doctor's bank account, and there was not a signed vendor confidence agreement between the doctor and the bank, could the deposit be considered a violation? When news of these examples were revealed on the Internet, much time and money was spent by practices on experts to determine whether violations had indeed occurred, and the rules were not yet published. In the last example, a quick call to the bank in question would have answered the question as to whether a confidentiality agreement had been signed or was even needed.

The final rules for "Patient Privacy" have been published. It should be clear to those that have followed this process that the real affect of HIPAA is yet to be seen and felt. It is not inconceivable that additional changes will be made if breaches occur. In many ways it could resemble a leaking dike where every leak will result in greater costs.

Really, what lies ahead in HIPAA implementation is largely unknown. The truth is that patients want and deserve to have their health care information protected. We can all agree, I think, that the health care industry will be better off by standardizing electronic data transmission.

CHAPTER 12

TECHNOLOGIES FOR A MORE EFFICIENT OFFICE

The premise of this chapter is that today's practitioner is performing more sophisticated services for less revenue and that in delivering those services, control by outside entities is greater than ever, in many cases interfering with the traditional doctor-patient relationship. Every reader of this book understands this premise, but there is a second aspect that is often overlooked: A physician's business office must do much more, in a more sophisticated manner, for less revenue.

I've lost track of the number of procedures and services that can no longer be rendered at breakeven in many practices. With the increase in managed care contracts, many large and small group practices have created an additional job slot in the business office for someone to oversee managed care contracts. Have you ever wondered what response you would get during negotiations over a managed care contract if you suggested that they would have to pay for the additional personnel you will need in your office as a result of the contract?

This trickle-down effect of changes in the provision of healthcare services and reimbursement of services also affects the vendors that serve you, such as collection agencies. Having served as a national officer of a national trade association of those vendors, I can assure you that increment fill—taking business just to fill the time—does not build a healthy and supportive vendor. At the same time, keep in mind that as a business office gets stressed, the accounts that flow through to the third tier are less collectible, compounding the problem.

A doctor I know began a solo medical practice approximately 18 months ago, and although it immediately flourished, she is facing a decision on whether to declare bankruptcy. Her practice began with a contractual relationship with a number of managed care entities, and the reimbursement levels she accepted would not meet the definition of increment fill. She was popular and began admitting a fair number of patients to a local hospital. The hospital which was interested in creating a strong, long term relationship, gave her loans to help get the practice started. It appears that no one ever asked whether or not the contractual care contract she had could support the loans she was taking from the hospital.

Realizing that she would have to cut costs wherever she could, in an 18-month period, she utilized the services of at least three third party billing companies, each of which quoted a rate lower than had the one before it. Although it should have been obvious that none of them could have performed the services necessary to manage her receivables at the contingencies they had quoted, it appeared on the surface that she had done all the right things. After all, it is hard to envision a healthcare professional working hard 6 days a week and failing to earn enough revenue to cover his or her expenses.

Guidelines For A More Efficient Practice

Realizing that many readers of this book are operating the type of practice in which a number of patients are at breakeven or less, I felt that exploring some cost-cutting techniques resulting from advances in technology might be helpful. However, let's do it in the following context. If the business end of a practice has to do more work for less revenue, in other words, create a bigger workload for those who have to' capture the reimbursement in terms of hours worked and costs incurred, this had better be in a way that makes the practice more efficient. To start with, let's use the following list as a guideline of what we are trying to achieve:

1. Reduce duplication of effort.

2. Improve cash flow.

3. Reduce staff time.

4. Speed the process of diagnosing and treating patients in regard to the management of paper.

5. Improve response time to any question regarding the economics of the practice.

6. Consistently follow through on an evaluation of anything that will help perform any of the above functions.

Where To Start

For many practices the biggest question is where to start, yet a road map has already been drawn. timelines for the more efficient use of technology have been clearly indicated by vehicles such as electronic media claims (EMC), the submittal of claims electronically and the receipt of remittances electronically, and other functions clearly applicable to A/R management. Although dates have been clearly established for implementation of most of this technology, it is reasonable to ask, If they are not met, will they be forced on the practice through legislative methodologies or perhaps through additional punitive measures, as occurred in the past? The difference between submitting electronic media claims and submitting paper claims is massive when one considers the great variance in the timeliness of payment. Let's look at the evolution of EMC in the belief that the process will not only continue but accelerate.

Electronic Media Claims

In the early 1980s the concept of electronic media claims was developed primarily for the submittal of Medicare claims. Medicare carriers were witnessing massive increases in paperwork but recognized that many providers were already using some form of data processing to submit those claims. As opposed to having the provider produce paper and forcing the carrier to convert it back to electronic media, people recognized the benefits of having the provider submit claims electronically directly to the carrier since this would not only reduce the amount of effort and work needed to process claims but also reduce the clerical errors created by transferring data. Providers were slow to accept this concept in the beginning because there were numerous challenges, depending on the discipline of the provider.

However, as Health Care Financing Administration(HCFA), now known as the Center for Medicare and Medicaid Services (CMS), soon recognized, it was the only way to keep up. As a result, HCFA held out numerous enticements for practitioners who submitted claims electronically, and in a short time those enticements were converted to penalties to those who did not. By the late 1980s many carriers who were determined to get the participation rate in the eightieth percentile, offered a host of options all being directed at the same goal: getting rid of paper. In theory, those options allowed almost any provider to get on the bandwagon. In some areas of the country the carrier simply offered a PC and modem with an emulation on screen of the paper claim. Although this was not necessarily an efficient methodology for the provider, since every claim still had to be keyed in, it still helped advance the goal of the carrier. Over the last several years EMC submittal of Medicare claims has become a virtual necessity because those who use it have been able to reduce their payment turnaround for all Medicare claims by 2 or 3 weeks. With the advent of improved software, a provider can identify problem claims within the first few days of processing.

Recommendation

If your practice is not yet using EMC, call your Medicare carrier and find out the scope of services and methodologies that are available to you.

Clearinghouses

Obviously, if the rationale of submitting claims electronically was good for Medicare, it should be good for all third party claims. However, most providers do not have a sufficient number of claims for carriers to make EMC worthwhile. Also, each third party carrier has individual parameters for the submittal of claims, and it would be ludicrous to develop the individual software necessary for direct submittal by each one. Finally, most third party carriers would be interested in EMC submittal only if there were some assurance that there would be close to zero error factors on the claims that they would receive electronically.

As a result, during the past 15 years numerous clearinghouses have been developed both nationally and regionally. They accept EMC claims from the provider that are normally acquired through a nighttime download by modem to the clearinghouse. The clearinghouse, having invested heavily told dollars in front-end edit processes, has the capacity to join all claims for third party insurance regardless of the provider. In most cases a clearinghouse develops a very stringent front-end audit to ensure that all data necessary for the processing of claims are present. The charge is paid by the provider and normally is based on a set fee per claim which varies with the volume of claims submitted. Obviously, this service gives the practice quicker turnaround and a significant reduction in the number of claims rejected. It is something that should be explored if not already in use.

However, initially there were some challenges. Many providers found that their software would not interface with that of the clearinghouse. Although most software vendors have attempted to correct that situation, some software allows for interface with only one clearinghouse. The second challenge is that although many major clearinghouses cover virtually all the major carriers, sometimes they do not cover certain local, HMO, or managed care plans. Under optimum conditions, if a practice is going to total EMC submittal, all carriers should be covered. The end result is that from time to time a provider must select a large national clearinghouse for the majority of its claims and a regional clearinghouse for local claims. This of dual system can become a nightmare. Although a provider may gain by having a reasonable price per claim with the national clearinghouse, it can end up paying a significant price to the second clearinghouse because of lack of volume.

Competition in this area and pressure from CMS on software vendors will improve this environment in the future. Practices that use EMC submittal for all claims through in-house efforts or clearinghouses will have a significant improvement in cash flow, and many of the rules of thumb for gauging a practice's performance will be changed. An example of this, the A/R ratio (Chapter 1) is optimally 4. For many that ratio has dropped to 3 because of significant turnaround on all third party claims. Although this is noteworthy and extremely beneficial, it is by no means a guarantee. It takes a lot of tracking to manage EMC correctly. Many who have tried it have found it to be a data-processing nightmare. It should also be noted that there are practices whose claim volume is so low that trade-off between the cost of the implementation and the cash flow and accuracy cannot be justified.

Recommendations

1. If you are not using a clearinghouse to process third party claims, your first step should be to get a handle on the number of claims submitted by your office on a week-to-week or a month-to-month basis and the number of different carriers to which you submit. If you ever elect to go to such a process, you want to make sure that the clearinghouse you choose covers the majority of the carriers to which you submit.

2. If networking with your peers ever made sense, this is the time. Find out what they are doing and their success rates, so that you can avoid making the same mistakes.

3. If you are using software from a national company, find out what is available. Talk directly to other users to get a feel for what you're into. If this technology is beyond your grasp, it makes sense to talk to a third party biller about what it can offer.

The Electronic Information Highway And EDI

The items identified above are primary to the overall concept of the electronic information highway, which basically involves the ability to move data electronically. Although these processes have their own standards, they do not take into account a far faster moving force encompassed in the reports of the Workgroup on Electronic Data Interchange (WEDI), which grabbed the attention of the government and insurance companies as it sought a way to reduce the management and processing costs of claims. The WEDI was a group of healthcare industry leaders appointed in 1991 by the secretary of health and human services, Louis Sullivan, to determine the steps necessary for the healthcare industry to move toward the use of electronic data interchange (EDI). EDI is and will remain as a very hot topic.

Electronic data interchange can best be defined as the electronic exchange of data between computers through the use of a standardized format. EDI is done not only by standardizing the formatting of information but also by using a standardized language. In essence, two computers not only can "speak" to each other but also can automatically place the information obtained into the correct places or positions and produce a document or record. EDI is a concept that is being developed in many industries; the banking community, for example, has been using it for years in the automatic teller machines (ATMs). In the healthcare industry, it is just now being developed. In the future, it will allow an insurance company to obtain accurate information from another computer without having a clerk "key" in that information.

Transaction Sets, ANSI and DISA

In the world of EDI, electronic business documents are known as transaction sets. For example, in healthcare claim reporting, Transaction Set 837 represents a form of a standardization for claims. That transaction set was created by a committees that worked under the American National Standards Institute (ANSI). ANSI committees were developed for the purpose of setting EDI standards throughout the United States. These committees have been working under the direction of the Accredited Standards Committee, which is known as X 12 or ASC X 12. ASC X 12 operates under the direction of Data Interchange Standards Association (DISA), in Alexandria, Virginia.

In essence, every element of healthcare claim processing is broken into work groups to standardize the definitions and the data needed in a transaction set. These work groups include initial claims, coordination of benefits, remittance and explanation of benefits (EOB). As each work group progresses under ASC X 12, the end result will be a standard that will be used by all participants. Obviously, all the insurance companies in the United States are not going to change their software, but it is assumed that all will create what is known as translator software, a means by which existing data can be received or output in accordance with the ANSI standards.

Electronic Bulletin Boards

The concept of electronic bulletin boards has become vastly popular. However, an electronic bulletin board by itself does not constitute EDI because it allows for the transmission of data but does not create standards for that transmission. If a bulletin board system is large enough, a certain degree of standardization will develop because of the design of the software. Furthermore, depending on the number of different databases that may become part of the bulletin board, one might find oneself writing interfaces not just for the bulletin board but also for those that would choose to go beyond the standards created by the bulletin board.

EDI is a very sophisticated and potentially expensive method for creating total standardization in the healthcare delivery industry, ensuring that all facets of the industry are recognized, including healthcare receivables, sharing of diagnostic information, electronic bulletin boards, and CPU-to-CPU transmission of EDI. To understand how sophisticated this is WEDI, which started this process for healthcare, in its first report, set 1993 as the target date for electronic mail, which was to communicate information beyond the standard transaction sets. However, all vendors and participants were expected to use "CCITTX400 Open Messaging Standards." Now I don't know what that means, but I can assure you it wouldn't be present in a bulletin board system. One must not confuse the highway (electronic bulletin board) with the vehicle that creates the road signs (EDI).

The Cost Of EDI

The largest present concern about EDI is its cost. Although initially envisioned as a one-time implementation, a one-time adjustment, and a one-time cost, it has now become clear that to achieve EDI on an on-going basis, there will have to be constant change and therefore constant escalation of the cost. One has to be concerned about how practices that remain outside large integrated networks will be able to stay current at a reasonable price if EDI is mandated.

If a practice that is having difficulty adjusting to EMC, envision the difficulties that it will have with the full scope of electronic interchange. For example, the concept of electronic remittance for Medicare is just around the corner. In fact, electronic submission and remittances have been implemented by some entities as an enticement to get others to join, eventually leading to the elimination of paper. Once again, there will be a demonstrable cost to the practice for not staying current.

Recommendations

1. Look to a third party biller to process your insurance claims, if not your total A/R. Alternatively, use another form of outsourcing and leave concerns about technology to others.

2. Many healthcare benefit carriers, including Medicare, conduct informative seminars. Someone from the practice should attend as often as possible.

3. Consider joining an integrated network in which a management organization service will take over the entire practice.

4. Look to other alternatives. Remember that EDI is only technology and don't let it force us to change the healthcare delivery system.

Other Technologies For An Efficient Practice

From a technological standpoint, advancements in computers, software, and other medical office support systems are occurring so fast that what is new today can be outdated in a short time. Those involved in computerizing the medical practice are striving to develop new technologies to entice the busy practitioners who are computer-reluctant and have little time to stay abreast of these technologies. Today there is an immense variety of software for the medical office. There are seminars, handbooks, and vast amounts of material on these systems. As this book was intended to explore the economics of healthcare A/R management, we will not examine the computer programs available for medical office management, diagnosing, and the like. However, here is a brief look into several technologies that can lead to better management of you're a/R.

Coding Software

Unfortunately, some coding software products were developed primarily to find the CPT codes that would generate the highest level of remuneration. Known to fraud and abuse people as "upcoding," coding software has become extremely sophisticated. At the other end of the spectrum, however, numerous fine software programs help ensure that diagnosis and CPT code are compatible and rationale. Other elements of these types of software help the user select the most appropriate CPT code, assure accuracy by checking for human error, and weed out list coding, such as gynecologic procedure for a male patient. If nothing else, this type of software helps create consistency in a practice. If the individual who does the coding changes every 6 months, a practice's profile in the insurance industry is going to have some significant peaks and valleys. Because of rapid changes in codes, coding software keeps one current.

Tracking Software

Because managed care will continue to grow and individual contracts with providers will have more variables, software has been developed that can help a practice monitor managed care contracts. For example, this software can compare the remuneration paid with the terms quoted in the contract. Practices that have used this type of software, which is normally geared for large group practices, have been able to document significant variances to the contract terms and as a result have reaped significant additional payments immediately. However, once the managed care facility is aware that is being tracked, these variances usually come to an abrupt end. Tracking managed care payments is a process that is virtually impossible to do manually, yet it is a function that will be essential in this area. It is also the forerunner to the technology that will be necessary in the management of capitative care. Again, it requires significant management and technological advancement, but in the end it can help regulate a loss factor that cannot be controlled easily without it. The next time a piece of mail that refers to this technology comes across your desk, read it.

Pen Computing

The personal computer (PC) is a common feature in medical offices. In fact, it is fast becoming a necessity. The perfect medical office would have a computer screen and a keyboard in every office so that the physician could have diagnostic information and patient history at his or her fingertips. Aside from the cost of having a terminal in every examining room, most physicians are hesitant to use any type of computers in front of their patients because the patient might feel they were not getting the practitioner's full attention.

PCs are getting more powerful, smaller and more portable, and less expensive every day. New technology has been developed that is a hand held computer. Data are entered and received through the touch of a stylus, a penlike instrument. It is totally portable and allows immediate access to all types of information.

Advances in all types of software occur daily. There is a program available that can walk a practitioner through a standard physical exam. The practitioner enters information as the screen rolls, and a printed copy of the physical is available by the time the patient gets to the front desk, along with prescriptions and a bill. Of course, to improve the profitability of a practice, the office personnel must see that a bill is presented to a patient and but that the patient pays it.

Document Imagining

Document imaging refers to the ability to convert every piece of paper in a practice to an optical readable disk (an electronic filing cabinet) and then quickly retrieve it and reproduce it in its original form or transmit it by facsimile. The technology, once considered expensive and not necessarily effective, has changed dramatically in the last few years. It can increase the profitability of a practice and help it control it's a/R. Those that have implemented it have found massive savings in terms of reduction of file cabinets, less paper usage, time saved in retrieval, and better control. It has been accepted by most governmental bodies and in most courts as a permissible substitution for an original document.

The applications of this type of technology are manifold. The amount of space needed to store patient records can be overwhelming. Let's say a practice elects to convert patient files to diskettes through document imaging. Although the process can take some time, in the end the practice will have significantly reduced the file space needed for storage, the history of every patient's record will be instantaneously available, and there will be a simple method for updating each record. That by itself may be something to consider. Better yet, envision that same practice opening a second office. Patients can be seen at either office. Rather than having to pull patient files the day before appointments and shipping them back and forth, through the use of a viewer at another off-site location or even at your home, you will be able to recall all your records.

Another application is that document imaging onto diskettes will allow for off-site storage of all patient records if there is a disaster in the office. One of the exciting facets of this technology is the ongoing ability to update third party carriers with additional information without taking a lot of personnel time. With this technology, one would could recall information to the screen and have the capacity to fax it and document the fax, specifying the date and time when it was sent.

Other applications for this technology relate to keeping timely informational files, particularly for Medicare, on changes affect a practice. Document imaging can also be used to store information such as an encyclopedia, which would do much to keep a physician's staff informed. There are numerous other sophisticated uses of this technology, one of which would allow the user, during the process of scanning the document, to lift from the document certain key data and transfer them directly to his or her computer. For example, if one was getting readable copies of consulting slips from a hospital, a patient's billing file could be actually created as part of the document imaging process. Also, those who have spent time going through a Medicare audit will readily appreciate the time this would have saved.

Predictive Dialer

The predictive dialer was originally designed for telemarketing. It is a technology that a practice would probably not want to get into on its own but might consider as an outsourcing service. It basically allows a downloading of all delinquent patients to equipment that automatically dials a phone number until someone is reached. Although it requires personnel, its value is that anytime a person is using the machine, he or she is talking to individuals rather than getting tape machines, busy signals, or no answers. It can increase phoning productivity by 200 percent or more in terms of reaching the right party. If you have a backlog of old A/R that needs phone attention before being considered for collection, this is something to consider.

Zip Code Sorting Services

For the busy practice that sends out a large number of statements each month, one has to consider the cost of the operation not just in terms of personnel and time but in terms of space used for inventory. As you may be aware, the U. S. Postal Service allows generous discounts for individuals who send their mail Zip code sorted. This of course would require more staff time and in all probability would result in insufficient amounts of mail being directed to each zip code. A solution to that scenario is to use a service that will pick up an office's metered mail at the discounted rate. This mailroom service then incorporates the practice's mail with all its other user's mail and sorts it by Zip code. A savings of 2 cents per statement may not sound like much, but over the long run and in high-volume cases, it starts to make sense.

Outsourcing the mailroom

Large corporations and collection agencies have used the concept of outsourcing the mailroom. This can be done every day or several times a month. When one is generating statements, the process is often tedious and slow. Even if an office has a high-speed laser printer, the statements have to be hand inserted into envelopes and stamped or metered and then sorted by Zip code. A mailroom service does all of that. All one has to do is download a print file by modem to the mailroom company, which will print a statement in its office that looks identical to the one a practice would send. The company then stuffs the statements, into return envelopes which are identical to those of the practice. Suddenly you no longer need to have staff members stay after hours to stuff those statements and get them into the mail. Just as important, of a number of other tasks are eliminated. No longer do you have to worry about inventory or the space used to store it, since the company supplies the paper and envelopes. Obviously the company gets a good deal on supplies because of its high-quantity purchasing.

There is another version of this service that is attractive to practices with a high volume, such as emergency room medicine and radiology practices. Most outsourcing mailrooms also check the address and name to which you are mailing against a standard computer file known as NCOA which is a database of the U. S. Postal Service that includes all forwarding addresses. If they find a deviation, they will correct the address for you and inform you about the change. In addition, they will convert your to Zip codes to Zip plus 4 plus 2, which will provide for more accurate and timely mail delivery.

Personnel and Compensation

There appears to be a growing phenomenon which is found principally in large teaching environments. In this scenario, each department is allowed to create its own billing and A/R staff, provided that it offers the employees the same benefits received by other employees in the healthcare institution. It sounds fair and equitable, but review the following scenario.

It is a respected department, filled with some of the best practitioners in that discipline. As a result, it has treated many patients from many different states. However, the department has not effectively dealt with the changes it has been going through. In the recent months the managers have come to realize that they have a significant A/R problem and need to address it so that their budget will not end up in the red for the current fiscal year. They were hampered, however, by two distinctively different problems. First, the software they use does not allow them to clearly identify patients who are delinquent and need follow up. The estimate for upgrading the computer system is in excess of $200,000, and the job cannot be completed until the end of the fiscal year, which will delay their attack on the problem. Just as important, all personnel within the department are being compensated according to the dictates of the institution. Although undoubtedly they are all superior employees and should command the higher wage, there is little they can do to justify their existence in regard to the existing computer system.

As a result of these two factors, another factor has come to light. The collectibility that they have been able to create on their existing system from their existing A/R was at least 18 percent lower than what other organizations in similar disciplines and similar areas have experienced. Although the department has taken the first step toward resolving the situation by outsourcing its receivables over 151 days of age, it is a long way from where it should be. For numerous reasons that have been created over the last 20 years, this department wants to have direct control over its billing. A look at the larger picture shows that if the managers examine the cost of upgrading computers, the cost of personnel, and an 18 percent increase in the collection rate, they will see that their cash flow could be accelerated by at least three times what their outsourcing arrangement calls for.

Specialists in A/R Management

Many vendors are also specialists and their ability to lower the cost of operations while increasing collections should not be discounted. Each field of A/R management has its own national trade association, some of which were mentioned in Chapter 1. This doesn't mean they don't have any bad apples, but to get information regarding third party A/R cleanups or A/R billing, one might want to make an inquiry to the International Billing Association. At the same time, let's recognize that holding on to receivables beyond a reasonable period should lead to consideration of the use of a third party collection agency. If that's the case, contact the American Collectors Association or Medical-Dental-Hospital Bureaus of America.

Summary

The primary concern in any practice is the performance of appropriate healthcare services. This is invariably the number one priority. However, it is also important to do this in an efficient manner that is economically sound. Therefore, a practitioner must look at every available tool and technological advancement that may help keep the practice moving ahead in an efficient and productive manner.

The healthcare industry, like every other industry, is going through a lot of changes every day. It is wise to stay in touch, listen to fellow practitioners, and educate yourself about the new technologies. However, you should try to stay levelheaded and not be overwhelmed by it all. After all, practicing medicine is your primary job, and these technologies can interfere with that. New ideas and computer software programs are wonderful, but if a new technology doesn't improve the way you deliver healthcare services or help in the management of you're A/R, it probably shouldn't be considered.

APPENDIX A

COMPUTER SYSTEMS REQUEST FOR PROPOSAL

Part 1: Practice Profile

Downtown Orthopedic Associates, S.C., is a group of orthopedic surgeons consisting of 6 physicians with 2 offices and 20 additional employees. We currently operate on a pegboard system with an average monthly patient load of approximately 800. Currently, our accounts receivable total approximately $1,500,000 with approximately 5,000 accounts.

Downtown Orthopedic Associates is looking for computer hardware and software that will perform the following duties: post charges, payments, and write-offs; maintain a total A/R for each physician, both separately and as a conglomerate; provide monthly reports of those items along with an aged A/R and regression analysis reports; send out billing statements in weekly cycles; and generate CMS-1500 forms for both Medicare and other insurance claims with the ability to send claims electronically.

The system must be expandable to accommodate additional physicians and patients and must be able to be operated from both offices, with the possibility of adding additional offices at a future date. It is a priority that there be flexibility within the system for adding new partners without the need for a programmer.

Please send completed RFP and any additional brochures that may be available to the name and address below by November 20, 1995. If you have any questions, please call me at (813) 221-4455.

> Josephine Jackson, Admin. Assistant
> Downtown Orthopedic Associates, S.C.
> 4455 Main Street
> Valhalla, FL 33445

Part 2: Vendor Company Profile

Company name, address, and phone number:

_____

Owner of the company or CEO's name:

_____

Contact person/sales rep's name:

_____

How long has your company been in business?

_____

Are financial statements available if requested?

_____

How many systems of this type have you installed to date?

_____

If available, please give names and phone numbers of users to contact:

_____

Is your company the author of the software? _____ If not, who is?

_____

May we have access to the source code if needed?

_____

Is there any additional information we should know about you or your company?

_____

_____

_____

Part 3: Software Specifications

1. Do you have an invoicing system (posting a payment, credit, adjustment, or write-off to a particular charge entry)?

_____

2. Will we be able to set up separate files for each physician?

3. Can we set up a new physician file without a programmer?

4. Can the system produce a "family" bill if more than one family member is a patient?

5. Does the program correlate CPT codes and ICD-9 codes?

6. Does the system allow multiple locations?

7. Is a security code feature available to limit access to certain users?

8. What additional software is available with your system? Windows? _____ Word Processing? _____ Spreadsheet program? _____

9. Does the system provide an aging A/R?

10. Does it produce Medicare and other CMS-1500 forms?

11. Can the software print checks in case of refunds?

12. Does the system have internal help screens?

13. Is there automatic backup?

14. Does the system create a patient ID number automatically?

15. Can a patient's records be pulled up by any means other than a name or account number? Explain.

16. Does the system allow for work address numbers in addition to home?

17. On Medicare assignment accounts, does the system automatically write off the disallowed amount?

18. Can two people access the same account at the same time?

19. Will it automatically generate a secondary insurance claim after the primary insurance is paid?

20. Is there a daily balancing mechanism? _____ If so, explain how it works.

21. Does it offer a daily journal of charges, payments, and adjustments posted?

22. Can statements be customized?

23. Can the system automatically write off balances under $5?

24. Does the system offer monthly and year-to-date totals for each physician by each of the following categories: charges, payments, credit adjustments, and debit adjustments?

25. Can it produce the same reports for the entire practice?

26. What other special reports does your system offer?

27. What is the total cost of the software specified herein?

Part 4: Hardware Specifications

1. What hardware are you recommending for your software to run on?

2. Does your company sell this hardware?

3. Would we be required to buy it from your company?

4. Do you lease this equipment?

5. What is the yearly cost?

6. How many additional terminals are available, and at what cost?

7. What type of printer do you suggest?

8. Does the hardware have the capacity for remote office sites?

9. What is the warranty?

10. Do you provide modems, power surge protectors, and fax add-ons?

11. What is the total cost for the proposed computer and all auxiliary equipment recommended for this system?

12. Does that include delivery and setup?

Part 5: Training and Maintenance

1. How many hours of training are included in the contract?

2. What is covered in the training session?

3. Where will the training take place? In our offices? Off site?

4.   How many people can we have trained?

5.   Is retraining available for new employees at a later date?

6.   If so, what is the additional charge, if any?

7.   Is there technological support? Is it free of charge?

8.   Is there a toll-free number for the support?

9.   Are there any user groups using this software? If so, how can I get in touch with them?

10.   Who will provide maintenance for the hardware?

11.   What is the cost for such maintenance?

12.   Is a maintenance contract available? _____ What is the monthly cost?

13.   What is included?

14.   What is the charge for noncovered services?

15.   What is your response time for service calls?

16.   In the event of a disaster, are there any users within a 50-mile radius with the same configuration of hardware and software?

APPENDIX B

LICENSING REQUIREMENTS

ALABAMA	Privileged Licensed Section, Gordon Persons Building, 50 N. Ripley St., Montgomery, AL, 36160, (334) 353-7827, fax (334) 242-0770.
ALASKA	Dept. of Commerce and Economic Development, Div. of Occupational Licensing, Collection Agencies, Box 110806, Juneau, AK, 99811-0806, (907) 465-2695, fax (907) 465-2974.
ARIZONA	Financial Services, 2910 N. 44th Street, Suite 310, Phoenix, AZ, 85018, (602) 255-4421 ext. 129, fax (602) 381-1225.
ARKANSAS	State Board of Collection Agencies, 523 S. Louisiana St., Suite 420, Little Rock, AR, 72201, (501) 376-9814, fax (501) 372-5383.
CALIFORNIA	Secretary of State, 1500 11th St., Sacramento, CA, 95814, (916) 653-7244.
COLORADO	Collection Agency Board, 1525 Sherman St., Denver, CO, 80203, (303) 866-5706, (303) 866-5691.
CONNECTICUT	Consumer Credit Division, Department of Banking, 260 Constitution Plaza, Hartford, CT, 06103, (860) 240-8200 ext. 8202, fax (860) 240-8178.
DELAWARE	Secretary of State, P.O. Box 898, Dover, DE, 19903, (302) 739-4111, fax (302) 739-3811.

DIST. OF COLUMBIA Corporations Division, Dept. of Consumer and Regulatory Affairs, 614 H Street, N.W., Room 407, Washington, D.C., 20009, (202) 727-7278.

FLORIDA Securities Director, Dept. of Banking and Finance, Div. of Finance, Capitol Building, Tallahassee, FL, 32399-0350, (850) 410-9805, fax (850) 410-9431.

GEORGIA Secretary of State, State Capitol, Room 214, Atlanta, GA, 30334, (404) 656-2881, fax (404) 656-0513.

HAWAII Professional and Vocational Licensing Div., Dept. of Commerce and Consumer Affairs, Box 3469, Honolulu, HI, 96801, (808) 586-2693, fax (808) 586-2874.

IDAHO Bureau Chief, Dept. of Finance, P.O. Box 83720, 700 W. State St., 2nd Floor, Boise, ID, 83720-0031, (208) 332-8002, fax (208) 332-8098.

ILLINOIS Board Liaison, Professional Services Sec., Dept. of Professional Regulation, 320 W. Washington St., 3rd Fl., Springfield, IL, 62786, (217) 782-6742, fax (217) 782-7645.

INDIANA Deputy Communication of Collection Agencies, Office of the Secretary of State, 302 W. Washington St., Room E111, Indianapolis, IN, 46204, (317) 232-0093, fax (317) 233-3675.

IOWA Consumer Protection Division, 1300 East Walnut, Hoover Building, Des Moines, IA, 50319, (515) 281-5926, fax (515) 281-6771.

KANSAS Secretary of State, State Capitol, 2nd Fl., Topeka, KS, 66612, (785) 296-4575, fax (785) 296-4570.

KENTUCKY Secretary of State, State Capitol, Room 150, Frankfort, KY, 40601, (502) 564-3490, fax (502) 564-5687.

LOUISIANA	Office of Financial Institutions, P.O. Box 94095, Baton Rouge, LA, 70804-9095, (225) 922-2592, fax (225) 925-4524.
MAINE	Office of Consumer Credit Regulation, 35 State House Station, Augusta, ME, 04333, (207) 624-8527, fax (207) 592-7699.
MARYLAND	Commissioner, MD Collection Agency Licensing Board, Commission of Financial Regulations, 501 St. Paul Place, Baltimore, MD, 21202, (410) 230-6098, fax (410) 333-0475.
MASSACHUSETTS	Division of Banks, 100 Cambridge Street, Room 2004, Boston, MA, 02202, (617) 956-1500 ext. 151, fax (617) 456-1598.
MICHIGAN	Licensing Administrator, Collection Practices Board, Box 30018, Lansing, MI, 48909, (517) 241-9231, fax (517) 241-9280.
MINNESOTA	Commissioner of Enforcement and Licensing, Dept. of Commerce, 133 E. 7th St., Saint Paul, MN, 55101, (651) 296-7977, fax (651) 282-2568.
MISSISSIPPI	Secretary of State, 401 Mississippi St., P.O. Box 136, Jackson, MS, 39205, (601) 359-1350, fax (601) 359-1607.
MISSOURI	Secretary of State, 208 State Capitol, Jefferson City, MO, 65101, (573) 751-4936, fax (573) 526-4903.
MONTANA	Secretary of State, State Capitol, P.O. Box 20281, Helena, MT, 59620, (406) 444-2034, fax (406) 444-3976.
NEBRASKA	Administrator, Collection Agency Licensing Board, Secretary of State, 2300 State Capitol Bldg., Lincoln, NE, 68509, (402) 471-2554, fax (402) 471-3237.

NEVADA	Commissioner of Financial Institutions Div., Dept. of Business and Industry, 406 E. 2nd St., Carson City, NV, 89710, (702) 687-4259, fax (702) 687-6909.
NEW HAMPSHIRE	Secretary of State, 204 State House, Concord, NH, 03301, (603) 271-3242, fax (603) 271-6316.
NEW JERSEY	Div. of Commercial Recording, Dept. of Treasury, P.O. Box 453, Trenton, NJ, 08625, (609) 633-8257, fax (609) 530-8292.
NEW MEXICO	Director, Financial Institutions Division, 725 St. Michael Dr., Santa Fe, NM, 87501, (505) 827-7100, fax (505) 827-7107.
NEW YORK	Secretary of State, 162 Washington Ave., Albany, NY, 12231, (518) 474-0050, fax (518) 474-4765.
NEW YORK CITY	Commissioner, Dept. of Consumer Affairs, 42 Broadway, New York, NY, 10004, (212) 487-4444, fax (212) 487-4090.
NORTH CAROLINA	Special Services Division, North Carolina Dept. of Insurance, Box 26387, Raleigh, NC, 27611, (919) 733-2200, fax (919) 715-1156.
NORTH DAKOTA	Commissioner, Dept. of Banking and Financial Institutions, State Capitol, 2000 Schafer St., Suite G, Bismarck, ND, 58501-1204, (701) 328-9933, fax (701) 328-9955.
OHIO	Secretary of State, 14th Fl., 30 East Broad, Columbus, OH, 43266-0418, (614) 466-2655, fax (614) 644-0649.
OKLAHOMA	Secretary of State, State Capitol Building, Suite 101, Oklahoma City, OK, 73105, (405) 521-3911, fax (405) 521-3771.

OREGON	Collection Agency Program, Div. of Finance and Corporate Securities, 350 Winter St. NE, Salem, OR, 97310, (503) 378-4140, fax (503) 947-7862.
PENNSYLVANIA	Secretary of the Commonwealth, Dept. of State, Room 302, North Office Building, Harrisburg, PA, 17120, (717) 787-7630, fax (717) 787-1734.

Public Protection Division, Office of the Attorney General, Strawberry Square, Harrisburg, PA, 17120, (717) 787-9716, fax (717) 787-1190. |
RHODE ISLAND	Secretary of State, Room 218, State House, Providence, RI, 02903, (401) 222-2357, fax (401) 277-1356.
SOUTH CAROLINA	Secretary of State, Edgar Brown Building, P.O. Box 11350, Columbia, SC, 29211, (803) 734-2170, fax (803) 734-2164.
SOUTH DAKOTA	Secretary of State, State Capitol, 2nd Fl., Pierre, SD, 57501, (605) 773-3537, fax (605) 773-6580.
TENNESSEE	Tennessee Collection Services Board, Volunteer Plaza, 500 James Robertson Pkwy., Nashville, TN, 37219, (615) 741-1741, fax (615) 741-1245.
TEXAS	Legal Support Unit, Secretary of State, Statutory Documents Division, P.O. Box 12887, Austin, TX, 7871; 1019 Brazos, Austin, TX, 76761, (512) 463-6906, fax (512) 475-2815.
UTAH	Dept. of Commerce, Div. of Corporations and Commercial Code, Box 146705, Salt Lake City, UT, 84144-6705, (801) 530-6026, fax (801) 530-6438.
VERMONT	Secretary of State, 109 State St., Montpelier, VT, 05609-1101, (802) 828-2148, fax (802) 828-2496.

VIRGINIA Secretary of the Commonwealth, Old Finance Bldg., 1st Fl., Richmond, VA, 23201, (804) 786-2441, fax (804) 371-0017.

WASHINGTON Dept. of Licensing Services, P.O. Box 9649, Olympia, WA, 98507, (360) 664-1389, fax (360) 664-2551.

WEST VIRGINIA Dept. of Tax and Revenue, P.O. Box 2666, Charleston, WV, 25330-7666, (304) 558-8610, fax (304) 558-1990.

WISCONSIN Supervisor of Licensed Financial Services, Department of Banking, Box 7876, Madison, WI, 53707, (608) 266-0447, fax (608) 267-6889.

WYOMING Collection Agency License Board, Dept. of Audit, Division of Banking, Herschler Building, 3-East, 122 W. 25th St., Cheyenne, WY, 82002, (307) 777-7797, fax (307) 777-3555.

APPENDIX C

SAMPLE REQUEST FOR PROPOSAL

Section 1

Purpose of Request for Proposal

It is the objective of Family Medical Center (FMC) to maximize the collection of revenue from patient and third party payers for services rendered. It is recognized that it requires the expertise of external professional agencies in the collection of past due monies. This document therefore serves as a request for proposal of collection agency services.

Background Information

Family Medical Center is a private medical institution with eight physicians specializing in internal medicine. It has hospital privileges at Memorial Hospital and has been a viable corporation since 1982. It has a computerized billing system and employs 20 people.

Section II

General Terms

This solicitation is a request for proposal and does not constitute an offer. Neither FMC nor the proposer is bound to any commitment. FMC may award one, more than one, or no contract at all. The successful proposer will abide by the laws of this state and of the federal government.

Sealed proposals consisting of three (3) copies must be submitted to the party below no later than March 14, 1994 at 5:00 p.m. Submit the proposal to:

> Mary M. Smith, Office Manager
> Family Medical Center
> 1234 Main Street
> Hometown, U.S.A. 12345

Qualifications

Proposers should provide detailed information regarding the principal owner/manager's qualifications. In addition, brief resumes of key individuals who would be assigned to this project are required.

Section III

General Conditions

After receipt of proposals, FMC may request interviews and additional information. FMC shall not be responsible for any additional costs other than for services outlined herein or for any work which has not been authorized.

Award of contract shall be to the low *qualified* proposer(s) who meets specifications in the best interest of FMC. If the contractor fails to progress under the terms of the contract, FMC reserves the right to terminate the contract with thirty (30) days' notice to the contractor.

Contents and Format of Proposal

Interested and qualified agencies must submit their proposals in the following format, addressing each requirement described below:

1.   A Cover letter which introduces the agency and the name of the individual who will be the primary contact with FMC.

2.   A statement of Objectives and Approach. Agencies shall use this section to describe the proposed services and address all issues listed in Section IV "Specific Requirements." Use of forms letters, phone calls, and so forth should be included with examples appended to the proposal. Collection activities, including frequency of follow-up procedures, should be described in detail.

3.   The agency should identify specific staff members who would be assigned to this project, their level and duties within the agency's organization, and their years of experience.

4.   At least (4) client references with name, address, and telephone number of individuals who may be contacted. It is preferred that at least one (1) reference be of the same or similar specialty.

5.   Current financial statement of the corporation.

6.   A fixed commission fee quotation, including a dollar cap for account placement, must be provided.

Section IV

Specific Requirements

1. Upon receipt of new accounts from FMC, the agency must provide acknowledgment of such accounts to include the patient's name and address, FMC account number, last date of service, account balance, and date placed with agency.

2. Sample copies of all form letters that will be sent on behalf of FMC must be submitted for review.

3. Payments received within five (5) days of acknowledgment will not be subject to a commission.

4. FMC will report any payments that result form the agency's efforts that are paid directly to FMC on the day they are received and posted.

5. The agency will remit collections to FMC monthly by the fifteenth day of the following month.

6. With the monthly remittances, the agency will supply FMC with the following detailed reports: acknowledgment of new placements report, monthly remittance report, monthly adjustments and/or closed accounts report. The agency shall also provide status reports when requested by FMC.

7. The agency must have the ability to receive and transmit data on tape to and from FMC.

8. The agency is required to be bonded under the guidelines of the state licensing board and submit proof of the bond to FMC.

9. The agency will operate in a professional and courteous manner and within the laws of FDCPA and the laws of the state in which it resides.

10. FMC reserves the right to recall accounts at any time, for any reason, without charge, provided that no payment has been made or is expected to be received by FMC.

11. The agency shall have the right to refer accounts for suit proceedings provided that it obtains written permission from FMC.

12. FMC retains the right to have access to and examine the books, documents, papers, or records maintained by the agency related to the collection of FMC account balances.

INDEX